Conventional Cures & Alternative Remedies

for
Everyday Problems

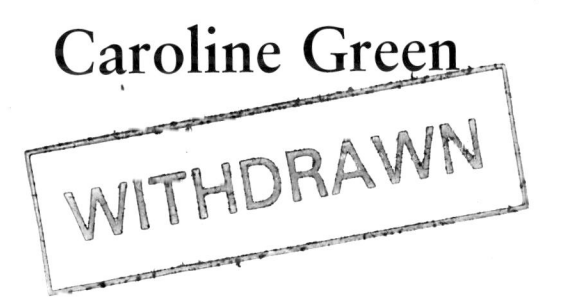

Caroline Green

MARSHALL PUBLISHING • LONDON

A Marshall Edition
Conceived, edited and designed by
Marshall Editions Ltd
The Orangery
161 New Bond Street
London W1Y 9PA

First published in the UK in 1998 by
Marshall Publishing Ltd

Copyright © 1998 Marshall Editions
Developments Ltd

All rights reserved including the right of
reproduction in whole or in part in any form

ISBN: 1 84028 142 1

9 8 7 6 5 4 3 2 1

Originated in the UK by DP Graphics, Trowbridge
Printed in Portugal by Printer Portuguesa

Project Editor Theresa Lane
Project Art Editor Helen Spencer
Design Assistants Philip Letsu,
 Michele Grigoletti
Picture Editor Zilda Tandy
DTP Editor Lesley Gilbert
Managing Editor Lindsay McTeague
Editorial Coordinator Rebecca Clunes
Editorial Director Sophie Collins
Art Director Sean Keogh
Production Nikki Ingram

The publisher would like to thank
Dr Penny Stanway for reading the text.

Note: The terms "he" and "she", used in
alternate sections, refer to people of both sexes,
unless a topic or sequence of photographs applies
only to a male or female.

Note
Every effort has been taken to ensure that all
information in this book is correct and compatible
with national standards generally accepted at the
time of publication. This book is not intended to
replace consultation with your doctor, alternative
therapy practitioner or other healthcare
professional. The author and publisher disclaim
any liability, loss, injury or damage incurred as a
consequence, directly or indirectly, of the use and
application of the contents of this book.

CONTENTS

Head & Chest Ailments

Headaches	8
Earache	10
Conjunctivitis	12
Styes	13
Toothache & Gingivitis	14
Cold Sores & Mouth Ulcers	15
Allergic Rhinitis (hay fever)	16
Sinusitis	17
Colds & Flu	18
Sore Throats	20
Tonsillitis & Laryngitis	21
Asthma	22
Bronchitis	24

Digestive Problems

Indigestion & Heartburn	26
Flatulence (wind)	27
Nausea & Vomiting	28
Reactions to Food	30
Diarrhoea	32
Constipation	34
Haemorrhoids	36
Irritable Bowel Syndrome	38
Food Poisoning	40

Aches & Pains

Strains & Sprains	42
Bursitis	44
Repetitive Strain Injury	45
Muscle Cramp	46
Neck & Shoulder Pain	47
Back Pain	48
Osteoarthritis	50
Rheumatoid arthritis	52
Gout	53
Chronic Pain	54
Chronic Fatigue Syndrome	56

Skin & Hair Problems

Cuts & Bruises	58
Insect Bites & Stings	59
Urticaria ("nettle rash")	60
Shingles	61
Blisters & Chilblains	62
Sunburn	63
Acne	64
Dermatitis & Eczema	66
Psoriasis	68
Corns & Calluses	69
Boils, Carbuncles & Warts	70
Athlete's Foot & Ringworm	71
Dandruff & Lice	72

Women's Health

Bladder Infections	74
Thrush	75
Premenstrual Syndrome (PMS)	76
Menstrual Cramps	78
Heavy Periods	79
Pregnancy Discomforts	80
Menopause	82

Children's Health

Nappy Rash & Cradle Cap	84
Colic	85
Mumps & Chickenpox	86
Measles & Rubella	87
Teething Problems	88
Emotional Conditions Stress	90
Insomnia	92
Depression	94
Anxiety	96
Panic Attacks	97
Seasonal Affective Disorder	98

Alternative Health

Alternative Health	99
Homeopathy	100
Herbal Remedies	102
Aromatherapy	104
Acupressure	106
Reflexology	108
Relaxation & Visualization	110
Acknowledgments	112

General Introduction

It can be worrying when you or a member of your family becomes ill, even if the illness is only minor. This book is intended to help you learn what can be done to treat the most common medical ailments. It will help you decide whether you can treat the illness at home or whether you should see a doctor or even call an ambulance.

Symptoms are listed for each ailment, and possible causes are outlined. In some cases, removing the cause may be enough to get rid of the symptoms; in others you may need more active treatment. You'll also find explanations of how a doctor might treat the condition. "See a doctor if" boxes give the symptoms that should always be reported to a doctor. If in doubt, however, you should ring your doctor's surgery for advice.

The book also provides information on alternative treatments, such as herbal remedies, homeopathy and acupressure, that can be followed alongside your doctor's advice. These are often intended to treat the symptoms and make you feel more comfortable; they are not intended to replace treatment by a doctor.

CHOOSING A PRACTITIONER

SEE A DOCTOR IF

- There is an unusual discharge or bleeding
- There is a marked change in your bowel or bladder habits
- A sore doesn't heal in 3 weeks
- A mole, freckle or blemish changes colour
- You feel a lump in your breast
- You have a nagging cough or hoarseness
- You have chronic indigestion or difficulty in swallowing
- You experience unexplained loss of weight or appetite
- You have recurrent vomiting
- There is unexplained severe pain, especially in the head, chest or abdomen
- You have a severe fever or night sweats
- You have unexplained fainting or dizziness
- You have blurred vision or see a halo around lights
- You have new or severe breathlessness
- Your lips, eyelids or nails have a bluish tinge
- Your ankles are swollen
- You have unexplained thirst
- You have weakness or unexplained fatigue
- There is yellowing of your skin or eyes
- As a man, you urinate often or with difficulty

FINDING A DOCTOR

If you do not already have a doctor, the best time to find one is when you are in good health. You will have the time to make a careful choice, and it will be easier for him to assess your health.

Ask friends and neighbours for a recommendation. Once you have a name, contact the doctor's surgery and ask about the doctor's professional qualifications. It is worthwhile finding someone who is part of a group practice. That way, if your own doctor is not available, you will be able to see someone else who has easy access to your medical records.

Before and after your first visit, ask yourself the following questions:

- Is the doctor the age and gender that you feel most comfortable with?
- Is the surgery easy to travel to?
- Can you get an appointment without much delay?
- Is the surgery clean and are the staff courteous?
- Did you have to wait long to see the doctor?
- Did the doctor take a full medical history and examine you?
- Did the doctor listen to what you were saying and take notes, and did he answer any questions that you had and put you at ease?

HOW CAN I GET THE BEST FROM MY DOCTOR?

Make sure you describe exactly what the problem is at the appointment. Don't expect the doctor to guess, and don't be afraid to ask questions. Make a note before your visit of things you would like to ask and take it along as a reminder.

If you don't think your doctor listens to you properly or answers your questions as clearly as you would like, tell him so. If communication doesn't improve, however, you may want to change doctors.

In certain situations you may like to seek a second opinion, for example if:
- Your doctor recommends surgery
- A rare or fatal disorder is diagnosed
- Your doctor does not make a diagnosis after several visits or tests and your symptoms persist.

CHOOSING AN ALTERNATIVE PRACTITIONER

Always see your own doctor before consulting an alternative practitioner for a health problem. Make sure the practitioner is appropriately qualified by contacting the professional body for the particular therapy. Otherwise, ask the same questions that you would ask your regular doctor.

Head & Chest Ailments

Health problems with symptoms that are experienced in the head and chest may result from infection or problems in one of several body systems. Apart from migraine and other types of headaches, of course, problems may include toothache, earache, a stuffy nose from a cold – which can cause blocked sinuses – and infections of the eye and mouth.

Many of these ailments, such as colds and flu, are the result of temporary infections and clear up of their own accord after some days. Your doctor may sometimes be able to prescribe drugs to cure these conditions, or may suggest rest and over-the-counter painkillers to relieve the symptoms. Many alternative treatments can also help. Long-term conditions such as asthma, however, may require more active medical treatment.

Headaches

Symptoms

Tension headache:
- A dull, steady pain
- Neck muscles may feel knotted
- Pain may be brief or long-lasting

Cluster headache:
- A mild aching feeling may precede an attack
- Severe pain around one eye, which may be red and watery
- Can occur several times a day for several weeks or months, with each one lasting from 30 minutes to 2 hours

Sinus headache:
- Pain behind the nose or in the forehead

Migraine:
- Severe, usually one-sided throbbing pain
- Nausea
- Visual disturbances

Causes

- **Tension headaches** are caused by tightening of the muscles in the scalp, face and neck due to stress or poor posture.
- **Cluster headaches,** which occur mostly in men, have many possible triggers, including smoking and alcohol, but the basic cause is unclear.
- **"Sinus headaches"** are caused by inflammation or infection of a sinus (see p. 17) or when nasal congestion partially blocks a sinus.
- **Migraines** result from constriction and dilation of blood vessels caused by a chemical imbalance with a great many possible triggers. ▶

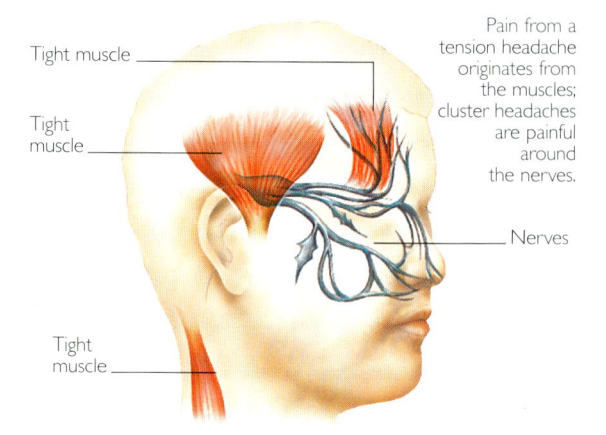

Tight muscle

Tight muscle

Tight muscle

Pain from a tension headache originates from the muscles; cluster headaches are painful around the nerves.

Nerves

Alternative Treatments

Acupressure

- You can relieve a headache by lightly pressing your middle finger between your eyebrows at the top of the bridge of your nose for 2 minutes.
- To relieve a tension headache, place the tips of your middle fingers in the hollows at the base of the skull on either side of the spine and press firmly for 1 minute.
- For a sinus headache in the forehead, place the tip of one finger in the bony notch a third of the way along the eyebrow from the nose. Press for 1 minute; release; and repeat 3 times.

Pressure point on the browbone between the eyebrows

Herbal Remedies

For migraine, chew 1 or 2 leaves of feverfew daily. Or take 3 125-mg capsules every 4 hours. **Warning!** Do not take feverfew if pregnant.

What your doctor would do

- Your doctor might suggest over-the-counter painkillers for a tension headache. You can also ask your pharmacist for advice on what to take.
- For a sinus headache, your doctor may also recommend a decongestant.
- Rest and relaxation will benefit those with tension or sinus headaches, as will applying alternately hot and cold compresses.
- Your doctor may suggest you avoid loud noises and bright lights if you have migraine.
- For migraines, your doctor may recommend one of a variety of drugs, in the form of pills, suppositories or nasal sprays, depending on the frequency and severity of the attacks.
- If you suffer from migraine, your doctor may advise you to stop taking the contraceptive Pill and to avoid any foods and beverages, such as red wine, cheese and chocolate, that trigger attacks.
- Relief from cluster headaches may require the prescription of a corticosteroid or other drug.
- Your doctor might take your blood pressure, suggest a vision test and, if concerned about other potentially serious causes of headache, might refer you to a specialist.

SEE A DOCTOR IF

- You have unusual or persistent headaches
- You have had a head injury and are drowsy, dizzy, nauseous or have vomited

Warning!
Get medical help immediately if a headache is accompanied by: vomiting; limb weakness; double vision; slurred speech; a rash which does not fade when you press the base of a glass tumbler against it; a stiff neck.

Aromatherapy
For a tension headache or migraine, blend a few drops of lavender oil into 2 teaspoons of sunflower oil and massage into the temples. For a sinus headache, use eucalyptus oil instead of lavender.

Homeopathy
Do not eat, drink or brush your teeth for 15 minutes before or after taking a remedy.

- For a sinus headache, try *Kali bichromicum* 6c every 2 hours, for 2 days.
- A headache aggravated by moving may respond to *Bryonia*. Take 30c every 10–15 minutes up to 10 times.

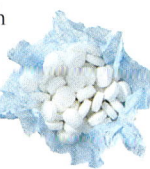

Bryonia

Reflexology
For a tension headache, apply pressure with the thumb to the base of the big toe. You can release the pressure after a few moments.

Reflexology point on the base of the big toe

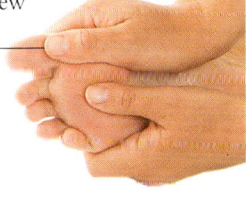

Earache

SYMPTOMS

INFECTION OF THE MIDDLE EAR:
- An aching or sharp pain inside the ear
- Fever
- Slight loss of hearing
- Discharge if the eardrum bursts

INFECTION OF THE EAR CANAL:
- Irritation or itching
- A discharge
- Mild deafness

EXCESS WAX:
- Sensation of fullness
- Partial deafness
- Irritated skin in ear canal

CAUSES
- An infection of the middle ear is the most common cause of earache in children.
- Middle-ear infection can result in a burst eardrum and a discharge from the ear. This relieves the pain because there is not as much pressure on the eardrum, but you should still see a doctor.
- If you swim often, bacteria may cause an infection of the ear canal.
- Excess earwax in the ear canal doesn't hurt but can be irritating. ▶

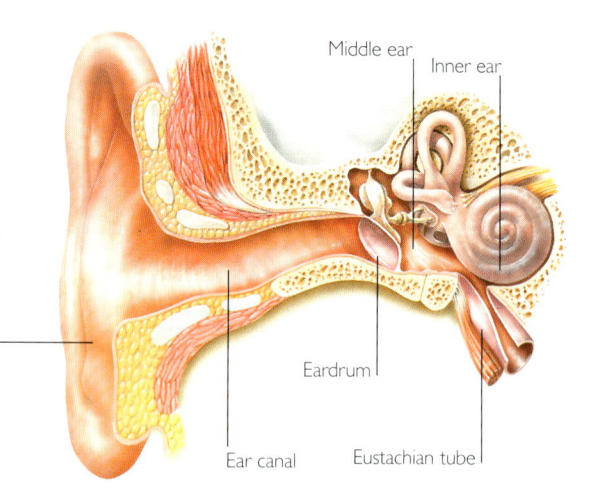

The pinna (the part that protrudes from the head) and ear canal are both parts of the outer ear.

Middle ear
Inner ear
Eardrum
Ear canal
Eustachian tube

ALTERNATIVE TREATMENTS

AROMATHERAPY
If the infection results from a cold, the cold should also be treated.

For a middle-ear infection, apply a hot compress soaked in a combination of chamomile and lavender essential oils floating on hot water to ease the pain.

To make the compress, sprinkle 4 or 5 drops of each of the essential oils into a bowl of hot water that is not so hot as to cause burning when touched. Fold a clean face cloth, handkerchief, or piece of towel or sheet and dip it into the bowl. Pick up as much of the oil floating on the surface as you can with the cloth. Wring out the compress before applying it to the ear. Alternatively, you can massage the essential oils around the painful ear.

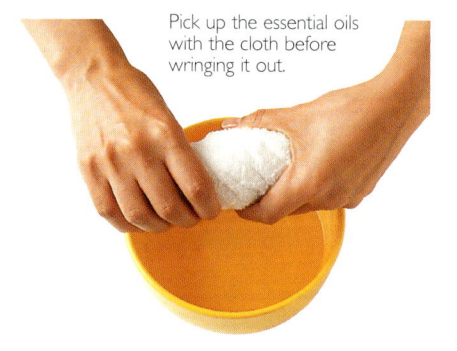

Pick up the essential oils with the cloth before wringing it out.

What your doctor would do

Your doctor will look inside the ear for an infection, using an otoscope, a special instrument that has a light on the end, and will examine the throat.

If there is infection in the middle ear, your doctor will probably prescribe antibiotics. Your doctor may also prescribe decongestant nose-drops to shrink the swollen lining of the Eustachian tube which leads from the middle ear to the back of the throat. When putting them in, lie back with your head turned to the side of the earache.

A discharge due to an infected ear canal may be cleaned.

Placing a covered hot-water bottle on the area may help ease the pain, as will painkillers.

Excess wax can usually be painlessly removed at home using commercial preparations. If you notice no improvement after three days, consult your doctor – who will use a syringe to flush out the wax. Because of the amount of water involved, this can be a messy process, but it is usually quite painless.

SEE A DOCTOR IF

- The pain is severe
- You have a high fever
- There is a discharge from the ear
- There is sudden or prolonged deafness

Warning!
Never insert any object in your ear, including cotton buds: they can puncture the fragile eardrum. If an object is lodged in your ear, have it removed by a doctor.

Homeopathy

Homeopathic remedies can be used to treat the earache itself. But if the earache results from a cold, then the cold should be treated too. The instructions apply to all the remedies below. Take 1 remedy at 6x potency every 2 hours, no more than 6 times on the first day. On the following 2 days, take the remedy 3 times a day. Make sure the tongue is "clean" by not drinking, eating or cleaning your teeth for 15 minutes before or after taking the remedy.

- If there is severe pain and irritation that is associated with chills or dry winds, take *Aconite*.
- Take *Chamomilla* for severe pain, loss of hearing and irritability.
- *Pulsatilla* can be taken if the symptoms of the earache include a discharge and fever and if hearing is affected.

Herbal Remedies

To soothe an inflamed ear canal, place 1–3 drops of mullein oil in it every 3 hours.
Warning! First, ask your doctor to make sure your eardrum is not perforated.

Verbascum thapsus, source of mullein oil

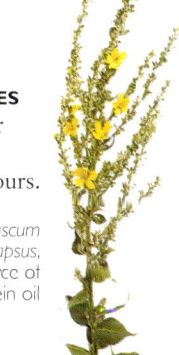

Conjunctivitis

SYMPTOMS

- Pain, irritation and a gritty sensation in eye
- Redness and inflammation of eye

BACTERIAL CONJUNCTIVITIS:
- Green or yellow discharge

VIRAL CONJUNCTIVITIS:
- Copious tears

ALLERGY-RELATED CONJUNCTIVITIS:
- Itching, and swelling of eyelids

SEE A DOCTOR IF

- The eye is no better after 24 hours

Causes
- Bacteria, especially in children.
- The viruses that cause colds, sore throats and measles.
- Irritants, including chlorine in swimming pools, smoke and dust, and allergens in cosmetics, pollen and animal hairs.

What your doctor would do
For suspected bacterial conjunctivitis, your doctor will prescribe eye drops containing an antibiotic. For a young baby your doctor may take a swab to identify the infection first. Conjunctivitis caused by a virus will disappear on its own. If an allergy has caused the problem, you'll be given eye drops containing an antihistamine or an anti-inflammatory drug.

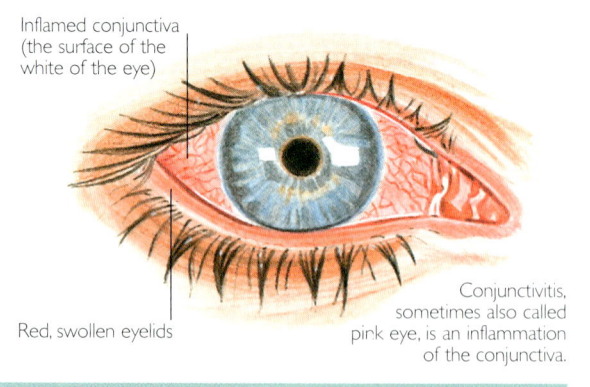

Inflamed conjunctiva (the surface of the white of the eye)

Red, swollen eyelids

Conjunctivitis, sometimes also called pink eye, is an inflammation of the conjunctiva.

Alternative treatments

Herbal Remedies
Try an eyebath. Put 1 teaspoon of dried eyebright or 2–3 teaspoons of dried chamomile flowers into 300 ml (1 pint) of boiling water. Simmer for 15 minutes and strain. Let it cool. Apply it to the eye with a clean piece of cotton cheesecloth 3 or 4 times a day. Store it in the refrigerator for up to 8 days.

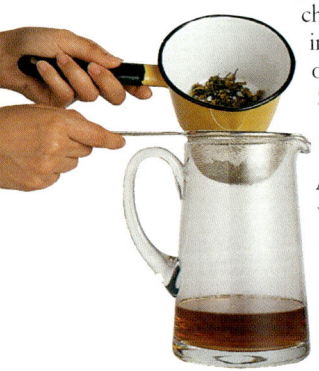

Homeopathy
Take one of these remedies 4 times a day for 1 or 2 days. Make sure the tongue is "clean" – do not drink, eat or clean your teeth for 15 minutes before or after taking the remedy.
- *Apis* 12x for red, puffy eyelids and stinging eyes.
- *Argentum nitricum* 12x for bloodshot eyes that feel gritty.
- *Pulsatilla* 12x for itchy eyes with a sticky, yellow discharge.

Argentum nitricum comes from the mineral silver nitrate.

Styes

SYMPTOMS

- Painful eyelid
- Redness and swelling
- Increased tears
- Sensitivity to bright light

OUTSIDE THE LID:
- After several days it will burst, then heal

INSIDE THE LID:
- A fluid-filled cyst can persist

SEE A DOCTOR IF

- The stye does not improve within a few weeks
- It interferes with your vision
- Styes recur often

CAUSE
- A bacterial infection.

WHAT YOUR DOCTOR WOULD DO
Styes often disappear after a few days and don't require medical treatment. A warm compress relieves the soreness and inflammation, and may help the stye burst. With your eye closed, apply the compress 4 times daily for 10 to 15 minutes at a time.

If styes occur frequently, your doctor may prescribe antibiotics. A cyst from an internal stye may have to be removed by a doctor.

A stye is a small, pus-filled abscess near the edge of an eyelid. It usually develops on the outside of the eyelid but sometimes forms on the inside.

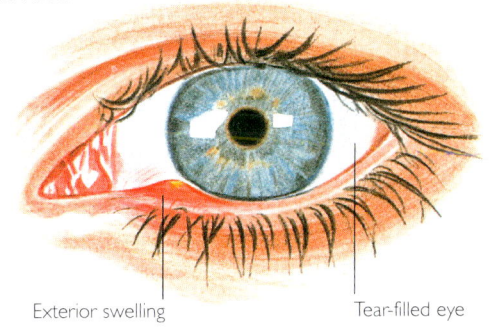

Exterior swelling — Tear-filled eye

ALTERNATIVE TREATMENTS

HERBAL REMEDIES
Eyedrops containing eyebright, made by a qualified herbal medicine practitioner, can help relieve the pain and inflammation.

HOMEOPATHY
If the eye is red, swollen and itchy take *Pulsatilla 6c* every hour for up to 10 doses. Do not drink, eat or clean your teeth for 15 minutes before or after taking a remedy.

Juice from the whole Pulsatilla plant is used.

OBJECT IN THE EYE

Try dislodging an object in the eye by blinking. If it won't budge, flush it out with clean filtered or bottled water. If it is still in the eye, gently lift the object out with a piece of moistened tissue. To see the object, you can lift up your eyelid by gently grasping the lashes, but first wash your hands.

Warning! If the object is difficult to remove, see a doctor immediately. Do not try to remove anything embedded in the surface of the eye or resting on the iris (the coloured part of the eye). Such an object must be removed by a doctor, usually under local anaesthetic.

Toothache & Gingivitis

SYMPTOMS

Toothache:
- A dull throbbing pain
- Sharp stabbing pain, which may be worse when lying down
- Pain when biting or chewing
- Pain when the tooth is exposed to hot or cold temperatures

Gingivitis:
- Bleeding gums after brushing the teeth
- Red, swollen gums

SEE A DENTIST IF

- You have a sharp or throbbing pain
- A tooth is sensitive to heat or cold
- Gums are red, swollen and painful

Causes
- A toothache is usually the result of tooth decay, although sometimes it is caused by a fractured tooth. It may also be caused by a sinus infection.
- Gingivitis occurs when plaque (a sticky deposit made of food particles, bacteria and mucus) builds up around the base of the teeth.

What your dentist would do
Painkillers help temporarily, but you must see a dentist for any toothache. Mild tooth decay requires a filling; more advanced decay or a tooth fracture may need root canal treatment, in which the pulp – the living tissue of the tooth – is removed in order to save the tooth.

Your dentist will treat gingivitis by cleaning the teeth. If the mouth is sore, gargling with a pain-relieving mouthwash may be recommended. An antibiotic is prescribed if there is an infection. You can avoid gingivitis by brushing and flossing your teeth daily, avoiding between-meal snacks containing sugar or other refined carbohydrates, and having regular dental check-ups. If left untreated, gingivitis can lead to more serious gum disease that can result in tooth loss.

Alternative treatments

Herbal Remedies
Oil of clove or myrrh rubbed on sore gums or on the gum around the painful tooth helps relieve the pain. **Warning!** Do not use clove or myrrh oil if pregnant.

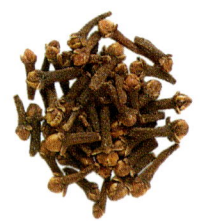

The flower buds and oil of cloves are used in herbal remedies.

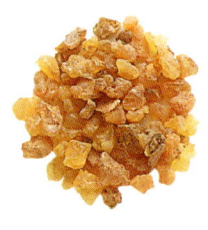

Myrrh is a resin from trees of the genus *Commiphora*.

Acupressure
To relieve the pain of toothache, apply pressure to the depression to the side of the ankle bone on the inside of either leg for up to a minute. **Warning!** Do not do this if you are pregnant, as it can induce labour.

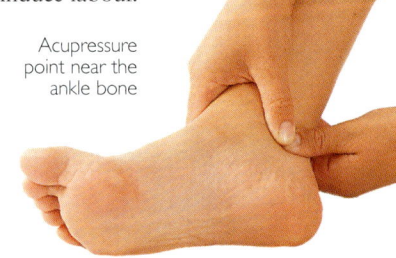

Acupressure point near the ankle bone

Cold Sores & Mouth Ulcers

Symptoms

Cold sores:
- Small red, painful blisters
- A burning or tingling sensation up to 24 hours before the sores appear

Mouth ulcers:
- Small, painful, white or yellowish sores that last 5–10 days

See a Doctor If

- A cold sore in the mouth doesn't go away after a few days
- A cold sore develops near an eye
- Mouth ulcers are recurrent

Cold sores are small blisters that are usually found around the mouth, but they can occur on other parts of the body. Mouth ulcers are painful sores that develop inside the mouth.

Causes

- Cold sores are caused by the contagious *Herpes simplex* virus. Some people have an outbreak once, others have them repeatedly. Stress, colds, menstruation and tiredness can trigger an outbreak.
- Mouth ulcers occur more often in adolescents and in women before their monthly menstruation. They may be triggered by stress or allergy.

What Your Doctor Would Do

There is no permanent cure for cold sores, but cream from a pharmacy reduces the pain. The doctor may prescribe an antiviral drug to help them heal faster. The viruses are highly contagious. To avoid spreading them on yourself or to others don't touch a sore. If you accidently do, wash your hands well immediately. Don't kiss anyone when you have a cold sore, and don't share towels or razors.

Mouth ulcers can be treated with antiseptic mouthwashes or ointments available from a pharmacist. Applying a cold, wet tea bag can help.

Alternative Treatments

Aromatherapy
To relieve either cold sores or ulcers, apply tea tree essential oil to the affected area, using a cotton bud.

Reflexology
For a cold sore, press the top of the big toe, the face reflexology point, for a minute. Then apply pressure in the same position on the other toes, which relate to the teeth.

Reflexology point at top of big toe, just below the nail

Visualization
To reduce stress, close your eyes and for 15 minutes imagine yourself in a peaceful place such as on a deserted beach or in the woods by a waterfall. Lying down helps, but you can also do this in a sitting position.

Listening to a tape of natural sounds can help you relax during visualization.

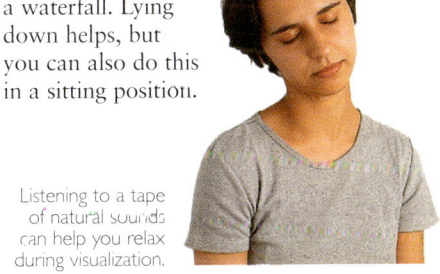

ALLERGIC RHINITIS (HAY FEVER)

SYMPTOMS

- A stuffy, runny nose
- Sneezing
- Headache
- Sore, watery, red eyes

SEE A DOCTOR IF

- You are uncertain what over-the-counter remedy to take
- Your symptoms worsen for no apparent reason

Sometimes certain substances trigger an exaggerated response in the immune system, causing the lining of the nose to become inflamed. This is known as allergic rhinitis, and hay fever – allergy to pollen – is just one type.

Causes
- Airborne pollen from flowers, grass and trees causes hay fever.
- Other types of allergic rhinitis are caused by certain substances such as animal hair, feathers, dust mites, air pollution and chemicals contained in hairspray or perfume.

What your doctor would do
The best course of action is to avoid the allergy trigger, although this is not always possible. Feather-free pillows and hypoallergenic cosmetics are available, as are vacuum cleaners with special filtration systems to remove the dust mites which are common in most modern homes.

Various over-the-counter treatments, such as antihistamines and sodium cromoglycate, can provide relief. Because prolonged use of some nasal sprays and drops available from a pharmacy can damage the lining of the nose, seek advice from your doctor if your symptoms persist.

ALTERNATIVE TREATMENTS

AROMATHERAPY
Inhaling the steam from 300 ml (1 pint) of very hot water containing a few drops of eucalyptus and peppermint oils eases sore sinuses. Or mix a few drops of lavender in a base of sweet almond oil and massage as shown, right.

Massage nose, cheeks and forehead with a few drops of lavender oil in almond oil.

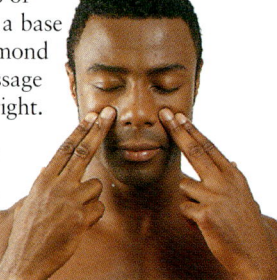

HOMEOPATHY
For runny eyes and sneezing, try 6c of *Allium cepa* or *Arsenicum album* as often as you feel the need, for up to 10 doses.

ACUPRESSURE
- Press the web of skin between the thumb and index finger for one minute. Repeat with the other hand. **Warning!** Do not do this if you are pregnant.

Acupressure point at the web of the hand

Sinusitis

SYMPTOMS

- Headache
- Sore, stuffy nose
- Thick nasal discharge
- Your face may hurt and feel "full" when you lean forward

SEE A DOCTOR IF

- Symptoms do not improve in 7 days or if they recur more than 3 times in a year
- You develop an eye inflammation

Sinusitis is an inflammation or infection of the membranes lining the sinuses, which are the air-filled spaces in the bones surrounding the nose.

Causes

- The result of nasal inflammation, often caused by a cold or flu.
- Hay fever and other allergies can sometimes bring on sinusitis.

What your doctor would do

Your doctor will probably recommend antibiotics, decongestants and steam inhalations. In severe cases, or when sinusitis recurs frequently, you may need to have surgery to improve drainage from the sinuses.

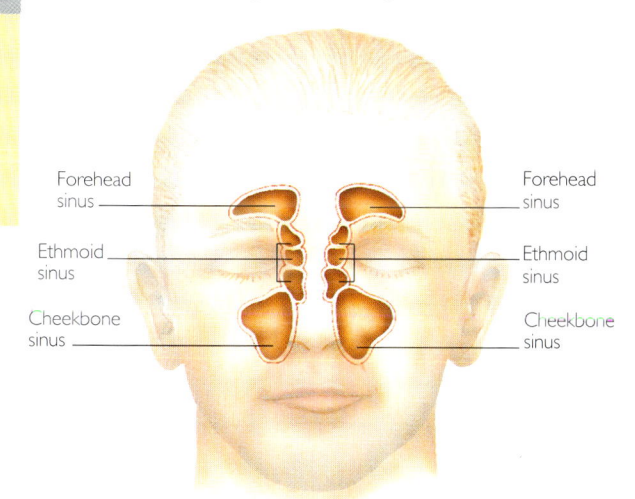

Forehead sinus
Ethmoid sinus
Cheekbone sinus

Alternative Treatments

Homeopathy

For a clear discharge, headache, sneezing and stuffy nose at night, try *Nux vomica*. Take 30c twice daily. Do not eat, drink or clean your teeth for 15 minutes before or after taking a remedy.

Reflexology

Apply pressure to the top and sides of the toes.

Reflexology points are at the top and sides of the toes.

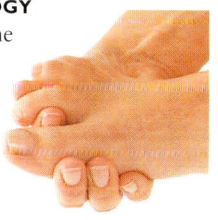

NOSEBLEEDS

Nosebleeds are caused by a blow to the nose, fragile blood vessels or removing encrusted material after a cold. To stop a nosebleed, sit up and lean slightly forward with your mouth open – this keeps blood from blocking the airways. Pinch the top of your nostrils and breathe through your mouth for 10 minutes. Release the nostrils slowly; do not blow your nose for 24 hours. If the bleeding doesn't stop after 20 minutes, get medical help. **Warning:** If the nosebleed follows a blow to the head, get medical help immediately.

Colds & Flu

Symptoms

Cold:
- Blocked nose
- Headache
- Sore throat
- Watery eyes
- Cough – tickly, dry or phlegmy

Flu:
- Any or all of the above, plus:
- Aching muscles and joints
- Fever

Almost everyone has experienced both the common cold and influenza, or flu. The problem is that it is often difficult to know if you have a bad cold or flu. The simple answer is that you'll feel much worse if you have flu.

Causes

Both colds and flu are contagious viral infections that attack the air passages; flu attacks other parts of the body too. You can catch either complaint by breathing in virus-infected air – in other words, being near an infected person who has just sneezed or coughed – or simply by shaking hands with them.

Contrary to popular belief, you do not catch cold from being caught in the rain, going outside without a hat on or sitting in a draft. Colds are most common in winter not because of the weather but because people tend to spend more time indoors in close proximity with each other and breathing hot, dry air. Children seem to be more susceptible to colds partly because a crowded classroom is an ideal place for viruses to be passed around and partly because they have not yet built up the resistance to the many cold viruses that many adults develop.

Alternative Treatments

Homeopathy

Do not eat, drink or clean your teeth for 15 minutes before or after taking a remedy.
- *Allium cepa* and *Nux vomica* are good for colds: take 6c every 4 hours for up to 10 doses.
- For flu, try *Aconite* or *Gelsemium:* take 30c every 2 hours, up to 10 doses.

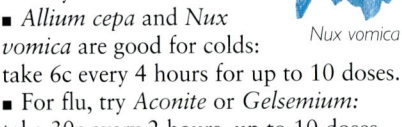

Nux vomica

Herbal Remedies

- Garlic can shorten the time you are ill; you can eat it raw or take capsules.
- An infusion of elderflower, peppermint and yarrow may help with muscle and joint pains. Add 1 cup of boiling water to 1–2 teaspoons of dried herbs. Steep for 10 minutes; then strain and drink.

Acupressure

To relieve coughing, bend your left elbow and make a fist, then place your right thumb on the crease of the elbow. Press firmly for 1 minute and repeat on the other arm. Do this 3 times.

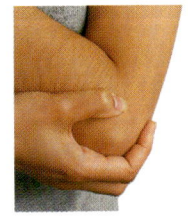

Point near elbow

WHAT YOUR DOCTOR WOULD DO

Once you become ill there are no drugs that will cure a cold or flu – you'll have to let the disease take its course. A cold normally clears up in a week or so; flu symptoms are usually past their worst after 2 to 5 days, but you may feel tired and weak for some time afterward. There are ways to ease the symptoms:

- Keep warm and drink lots of liquids, especially water and fresh fruit juice.
- Take over-the-counter painkillers to help ease headaches and joint or muscle pain.
- Use decongestants to clear a blocked nose. Don't take them for more than 5 days as prolonged use can make the stuffiness worse. They can also make you drowsy, so don't take them if you have to drive or operate machinery.
- Over-the-counter cough medicines can help in the short term, but they only suppress the urge to cough – they don't cure it. Use them for night-time relief only, and not longer than 7–10 days. Drinking a lot of water can help loosen phlegm as much as an expectorant cough syrup does.

Vaccinations against flu are available, but are not 100 percent successful. They are generally given annually and are especially recommended for the elderly and people with certain chronic illnesses.

SEE A DOCTOR IF

- Your cough lasts more than a week
- A fever lasts longer than 3 days, or if symptoms include a severe headache, a stiff neck, abdominal pain or pain passing urine
- The person suffering from a high fever is a baby under 6 months old, an elderly person, or a child with a history of convulsions

Warning!
If a cough is accompanied by a high fever, difficulty in breathing, blue tongue or lips, drowsiness or difficulty in speaking, call a doctor at once.

AROMATHERAPY

Steam inhalations of menthol, eucalyptus or peppermint oil help clear a blocked nose. Pour a few drops into a basin of very hot water, cover your head with a towel and breathe in the vapour for 5 minutes or so.

A steam inhalation can clear a blocked nose.

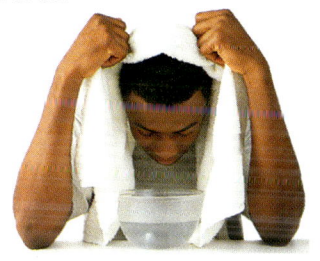

FEVERS

A fever is a temperature above 38°C (100°F) and is a common symptom of flu and many other illnesses. It may be accompanied by shivering, sweating, headache, thirst and flushed skin.

Many over-the-counter painkillers – such as aspirin or paracetamol – help relieve a fever. If you have a bacterial infection, your doctor may prescribe antibiotics. Drink plenty of fluids to replace those through sweating. Do not wear too many clothes or bedclothes or have the room too hot.
Warning! Never give aspirin to a child under 12 years of age.

Sore Throats

SYMPTOMS

- Irritation, a tickling sensation, a feeling of heat or "rawness" at the back of the throat
- Visible redness at the back of the throat
- Tenderness in the neck

STREP THROAT:
- Back of the throat is very painful
- A fever above 39°C (101°F)

SEE A DOCTOR IF

- A sore throat or fever lasts more than a few days
- A fever rises high, especially in a baby
- You have trouble breathing or swallowing

The expression "sore throat" is self-explanatory and almost everyone gets one from time to time. Usually sore throats are not much more than an irritation, but occasionally they can be serious and require medical treatment.

CAUSES

- Viral infections, such as colds, flu and chickenpox, can cause a sore throat.
- Bacterial infections, including whooping cough, can lead to a sore throat. One type of bacteria – beta-haemolytic streptococci – can cause a "strep throat", a severe sore throat that, if left unchecked, occasionally has serious complications.

WHAT YOUR DOCTOR WOULD DO

Most sore throats clear up by themselves. To ease the soreness, you can gargle with an antiseptic solution, rest and drink plenty of fluids (though avoid carbonated drinks, which can irritate the throat). Using a humidifier in your bedroom will help to keep your throat moist.

If your doctor suspects that you have a bacterial infection, he may take a swab from your throat and send it to a laboratory to be tested for bacteria. If necessary, your doctor will prescribe antibiotics.

ALTERNATIVE TREATMENTS

HOMEOPATHY
Belladonna and *Aconite* are commonly recommended. Use either remedy in the 30c potency and take it every 2 hours for up to 10 doses.

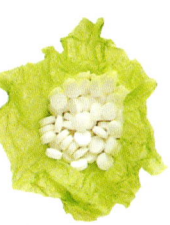

Belladonna

HERBAL REMEDIES
Garlic, either in capsules or raw, boosts the immune system, keeping infection at bay. Alternatively, try sage, chamomile or liquorice tea to soothe a sore throat.
Warning! Avoid sage tea if pregnant.

ACUPRESSURE
- Press your left thumb on the middle of the pad at the base of your right thumb for 1 minute and release. Repeat on the other hand.
- Using your thumb, press the sole of your foot in the depression under the ball of the foot for 1 minute.

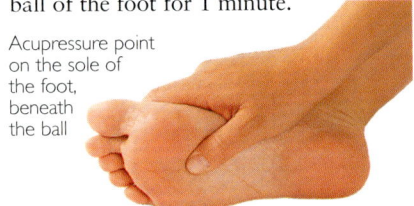

Acupressure point on the sole of the foot, beneath the ball

Tonsillitis & Laryngitis

Causes
- Cold or flu viruses or the same bacteria that can cause a "strep throat" can cause tonsillitis.
- Laryngitis may be caused by a viral or bacterial infection, allergy, breathing in chemical vapour, or overusing your voice.

What your doctor would do
In both cases your doctor may recommend bed rest with plenty of fluids, and over-the-counter painkillers if necessary. You may also be given antibiotics for a bacterial infection or antihistamines for an allergy.

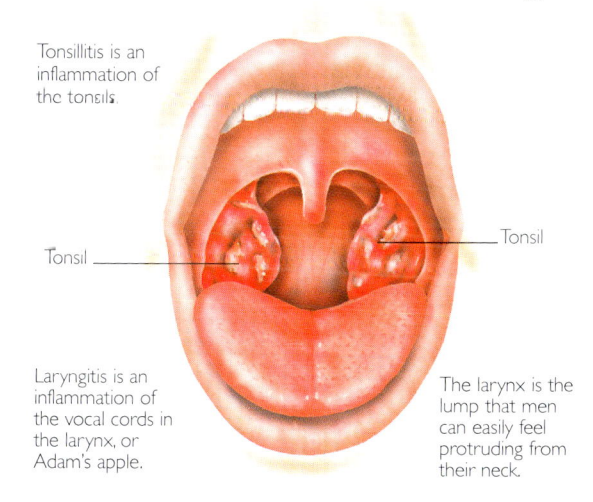

SYMPTOMS

Tonsillitis:
- Sore throat
- Hard to swallow
- Fever
- Spots on the tonsils or a white discharge
- Headache

Laryngitis:
- Hoarseness
- Loss of voice
- Sore throat
- Fever
- Cough

Tonsillitis is an inflammation of the tonsils.

Tonsil

Tonsil

Laryngitis is an inflammation of the vocal cords in the larynx, or Adam's apple.

The larynx is the lump that men can easily feel protruding from their neck.

SEE A DOCTOR IF
- A sore throat lasts more than a few days
- Hoarseness lasts more than one week
- You cough up phlegm

Alternative Treatments

Herbal Remedies
Elderflower taken as a tincture can help reduce inflammation. To prepare a tincture, half-fill a large screw-topped jar with the chopped or ground herb, fill the jar with alcohol (vodka is ideal) and store in a warm place away from direct sunlight. Shake the jar twice a day. After 2 weeks, decant the mixture into another jar and store in a cool place. Take 10–30 drops straight or mixed with water, up to 4 times a day.

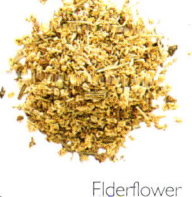

Elderflower

- Or, gargle with warm tea made from red sage, bayberry or white oak. Steep 1–2 teaspoons of the herb in a cup of hot water for 10 minutes and strain. Gargle with it several times a day. **Warning!** Do not use sage gargles if pregnant.

Homeopathy
Spongia helps a dry throat, while *Aconite* is useful in the early stages of a cold with laryngitis. Take either remedy in 30c potency every 2 hours for up to 10 doses. Do not eat, drink or clean your teeth for 15 minutes before or after taking either one.

Asthma

SYMPTOMS

- Wheezing
- A feeling of tightness in the chest
- Shortness of breath
- A cough, which may be dry or phlegmy
- Symptoms may be mild or severe

Causes
- The most common cause is an allergic reaction to one or more of several possible trigger substances, including animal hair, house dust, tobacco smoke, certain foods and over-the-counter drugs such as aspirin. Allergy-related asthma is often hereditary.
- Asthma may be brought on by stress, exercise and air pollution.
- Lung infections can also cause asthma. ▶

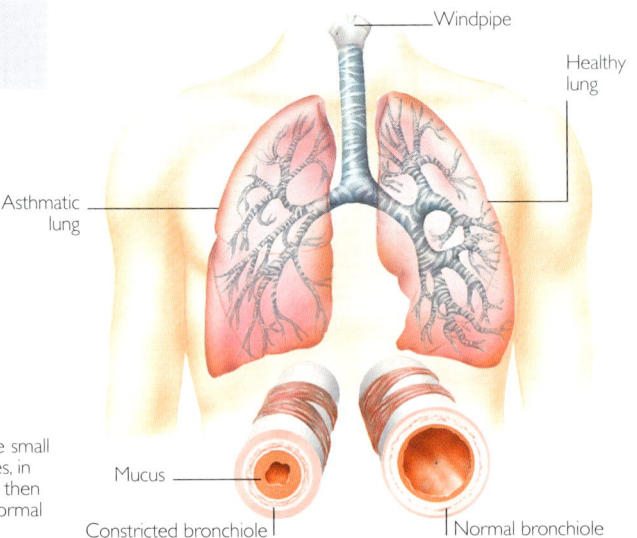

In people with asthma, the small air passages, or bronchioles, in the lungs constrict. Mucus then builds up and obstructs normal breathing.

Windpipe
Healthy lung
Asthmatic lung
Mucus
Constricted bronchiole
Normal bronchiole

Alternative treatments

Acupressure
Try either of these pressure points if you think an asthma attack is about to start:
- Press your thumb at the acupressure point 2 fingers' width from the wrist crease nearest the palm, on the inside of the forearm and in line with the thumb.
- Reach around behind your head and press each thumb gently on the acupressure points that are about a finger's width away from each side of the spine.

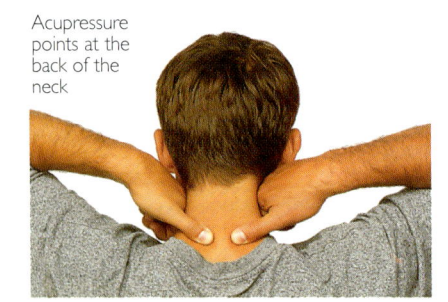

Acupressure points at the back of the neck

Homeopathy
A trained homeopath will recommend various treatments for asthma, depending on the individual. Here are a few you can try yourself:

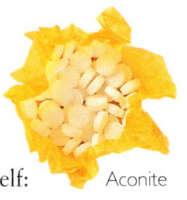

Aconite

What your doctor would do

First your doctor will try to help you establish what triggers your asthma. If you don't know what brings it on, you may need to keep a diary so that you and your doctor can work out what is most likely to be the trigger. You will then be given advice on ways of eliminating the triggers or reducing their effect.

You may be prescribed a drug known as a bronchodilator, which helps open the narrowed airways in the lungs. This will either be taken by mouth or from an inhaler. If your asthma is serious, your doctor may also prescribe a corticosteroid – a drug similar to a natural hormone in the body – which is useful both in preventing symptoms and as an emergency treatment for an attack.

If you smoke, your doctor will strongly recommend that you stop immediately. He may also help you learn how to cope better with stress.

> **SEE A DOCTOR IF**
>
> - It is the first time you have had an attack
> - Any drugs do not work as soon as they should – you may need new ones

> **Warning!**
> Call for emergency help right away if an asthmatic person complains of a suffocating feeling and finds it hard to talk; their nostrils flare; the skin between their ribs looks pulled in; and their nails or lips look bluish. This means they can't breathe in enough oxygen or breathe out enough carbon dioxide.

Arsenicum album, take 30c as required; *Aconite*, 6c when needed; and *Natrum sulphuricum*, 6c when needed. Do not eat, drink or clean your teeth for 15 minutes before or after taking a remedy.

Herbal Remedies

An infusion from the root of elecampane may help a phlegmy chest. An infusion of mullein is good at night time. To prepare an infusion, steep a herbal tea-bag or a teaspoon of the dried herb in a cup of boiling water for 5 minutes (then strain, if using dried herbs). You can add honey if you like.

Reflexology

You may find some relief from asthma by applying pressure with your thumb on the lower part of the ball of foot. You can find the point by following an imaginary line down from between the big toe and its neighbouring toe (the toes here are spread apart for clarity).

Reflexology point below the ball of the foot

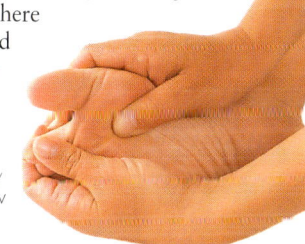

Bronchitis

Symptoms

Acute bronchitis:
- A hacking cough
- White, yellow or green phlegm
- Fever
- A sore, tight chest
- Pain when breathing deeply

Chronic bronchitis:
- A cough that persists for 3 months at a time
- White, yellow or green phlegm

Call a Doctor if

- A cough persists for more than a week
- Your cough produces white, yellow or green phlegm
- You experience breathing difficulties

Bronchitis develops when the airways that connect the windpipe to the lungs become inflamed. There are two kinds: acute and chronic. Acute bronchitis is usually less serious and shouldn't last for more than two weeks, but it can be dangerous in elderly people and in those who have had a heart attack. Chronic bronchitis is more serious and may last for months.

Causes

- A viral infection is the most common cause of acute bronchitis, although bacteria are responsible in 10 percent of people.
- Chronic bronchitis may develop in people who have repeated bouts of acute bronchitis.
- Industrial pollution and repeated exposure to dust can also cause chronic bronchitis, as can long-term heavy cigarette smoking.

What your doctor would do

For acute bronchitis, the doctor may prescribe antibiotics or advise taking over-the-counter painkillers, resting and drinking plenty of fluids.

For chronic bronchitis, the doctor may recommend annual vaccinations to prevent flu, and a one-off vaccination to prevent pneumonia, or he may prescribe drugs to dilate the airways.

Anyone who suffers from either type of bronchitis is well advised to give up smoking.

Alternative Treatments

Homeopathy

Try one of these remedies every 4 hours for up to 10 doses. Do not eat, drink or clean your teeth for 15 minutes before or after taking a remedy.
- For a fever, cough and tightness around your chest, take *Aconite* 30c.
- If you have a hoarse voice, sore throat, cough and thirst, try *Phosphorus* 6c.

Herbal Remedies

- Coltsfoot can relax constricted passages and mullein may have anti-inflammatory properties. To take either of these, make an infusion by steeping 1–2 teaspoons of the dried herb in a cup of boiling water for 10 minutes, then strain. Drink the infusion while it is still hot 3 times daily.
- To boost your immune system, take garlic daily, raw or in capsule form.

Aromatherapy

To improve breathing, try inhalations of steam scented with eucalyptus, lavender, rosemary or hyssop. Pour a few drops of the essential oil into a basin of boiling water. Inhale the vapour for 5 minutes. Or put a few drops of oil on to a handkerchief and inhale. **Warning!** Do not use hyssop oil if pregnant.

DIGESTIVE PROBLEMS

The food you eat is processed in the digestive system, starting in the mouth. As you chew, your teeth grind the food into smaller pieces and saliva begins to break it down. It then travels through the gastrointestinal system: the oesophagus, stomach and small and large intestines. In each part of the system food is further churned and processed with a variety of enzymes to release vital nutrients before the waste is expelled.

It's a complicated system, which does not always run smoothly, and a variety of factors may cause problems. An infection can result in nausea or diarrhoea; alcohol consumption and smoking may trigger indigestion; specific foods cause allergic reactions in some people; and too much stress can have adverse effects. For each of these complaints there are a number of treatments to ease or cure the symptoms.

INDIGESTION & HEARTBURN

SYMPTOMS

INDIGESTION:
- Abdominal pain
- Belching or flatulence
- Mild nausea
- Vomiting

HEARTBURN:
- As for indigestion, but with a burning sensation in the centre of the chest, especially when lying down

SEE A DOCTOR IF

- Abdominal pain lasts over 6 hours or is severe or frequent
- You vomit blood or pass a very dark stool
- You feel dizzy, faint or feverish

Indigestion is a general term for various stomach problems brought on by eating; heartburn is a type of indigestion in which stomach acid enters and irritates the throat.

CAUSES
- Both complaints are often brought on by eating too much, too quickly, by eating rich or spicy foods, or by drinking too much alcohol.
- Being seriously overweight may cause either.
- Stress is also a cause of indigestion, as is smoking.
- Frequent indigestion may result from a bacterial infection associated with a peptic ulcer.
- Some pain-relievers can cause indigestion.
- A weak muscular valve around the gullet can lead to heartburn.

WHAT YOUR DOCTOR WOULD DO
Avoiding foods that cause problems helps, as does trying to relax when you eat, but if indigestion occurs frequently, you should see your doctor.

If there is no serious cause for your indigestion or heartburn, your doctor may suggest antacid tablets. But if you are in danger of developing an ulcer from the excess stomach acid that sometimes accompanies indigestion, she may recommend a medicine to coat the stomach lining instead. If a bacterial infection is to blame, she will prescribe antibiotics.

ALTERNATIVE TREATMENTS

HOMEOPATHY
For heartburn, take 6c of *Arsenicum album* 3 times at 15-minute intervals; you can repeat the series if necessary.

AROMATHERAPY
Massage is good for digestive problems because it can help the circulation in the stomach area. It happens to be a good way to relax, too, which is also beneficial for people with indigestion. The essential oils of bergamot, chamomile, fennel, melissa and peppermint are all good for aiding indigestion. Using light pressure, massage one of the recommended essential oils on the abdomen in a clockwise direction.
Warning! Do not have an abdominal massage if you have diverticulitis, Crohn's disease, ulcers, cancer or any other serious or inflammatory condition.

Abdominal massage stimulates circulation and can alleviate indigestion.

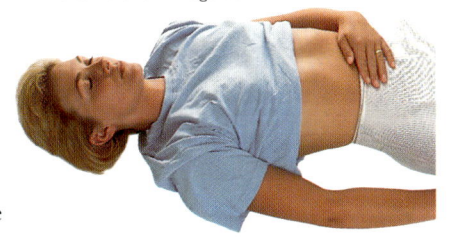

Flatulence (wind)

SYMPTOMS
■ A bloated feeling
■ A frequent need to burp or break wind
■ Abdominal pain

SEE A DOCTOR IF
■ Symptoms last more than 3 days: they could indicate an ulcer, hiatus hernia, irritable bowel or lactose-intolerance

When wind builds up in the body it needs to find a way out. This is normal and usually a minor problem, but in some cases it can be a nuisance and possibly lead to extreme discomfort.

Causes
■ Swallowing too much air when eating, drinking carbonated beverages, chewing gum, swallowing a lot when wearing false teeth, or feeling nervous can all cause wind.
■ Eating high-fibre foods, including pulses, certain other vegetables and fruits, can cause wind.
■ Wind can be a painful problem in people with lactose-intolerance who do not have the enzyme needed to digest sugar (lactose) in dairy foods.
■ Wind can also result from an infection in the digestive system.

What your doctor would do
You can usually relieve flatulence without consulting a doctor. Chewing food slowly and sitting up straight when eating meals helps, as does avoiding any foods and beverages that cause the problem. Over-the-counter medicines can break up the wind from pulses such as baked beans. Tablets and drops of lactase – the enzyme needed to digest lactose – allow lactose-intolerant people to eat dairy products.

Alternative Treatments

Acupressure
With the thumb and index finger of one hand, squeeze the web of skin between the thumb and index finger of the other hand; repeat on the other hand. **Warning!** Do not do this if you are pregnant.

Herbal Remedies
Chamomile and peppermint teas can soothe indigestion. Eating garlic, caraway seeds and cloves, and using thyme and marjoram in cooking, can also help. Garlic is best raw, but is available in capsules.

Hiccups

Hiccups are caused by spasms of the diaphragm, which lies beneath the rib cage. They may be caused by eating or drinking too much or too fast, or by drinking alcohol.

They usually go away on their own accord, but if they persist, try holding your breath, drinking water from the far rim of a glass or breathing in and out of a paper bag (do not do this for more than 3 minutes). Or try drinking a cup of lemon balm or peppermint tea.

Warning! See your doctor if hiccups last for more than a day.

Nausea & Vomiting

Symptoms

- Nausea is a feeling of wanting to be sick, not necessarily accompanied by vomiting
- A wave of heat followed by a cold clamminess often culminates in vomiting

Motion sickness:
- Sweating and dizziness, along with nausea, when travelling

Nausea is one of the commonest ailments and sometimes, but not always, leads to vomiting. Vomiting occurs when involuntary muscle spasms force the stomach to eject its contents through the mouth.

Causes

- Both nausea and vomiting can be caused by eating food that has begun to decay or to which you are allergic.
- People with flu or other infections may experience nausea and vomiting.
- A disturbance in your balance can make you feel sick or vomit. This often occurs in the form of motion sickness; when you travel by car, bus, boat or plane, what you see doesn't match up with what the balance mechanism in your ear senses and this has rapid consequences in some people.
- Nausea and vomiting is common in early pregnancy (see pp. 80–81).
- Two of the symptoms of migraine are nausea and vomiting.
- Certain serious complaints, such as hepatitis, uncontrolled diabetes, and appendicitis, can cause nausea and vomiting. ▶

Alternative treatments

Herbal Remedies

Try an infusion of ginger, Roman chamomile or black horehound to reduce nausea. Infuse a tea-bag or a teaspoon of the dried herb in a cup of boiling water for 5 minutes; strain it if needed.
Warning! Do not use black horehound if pregnant.

Ginger root is an old remedy for nausea.

Homeopathy

Take 12x dosages of either remedy every 2 hours as needed. Do not eat, drink or clean your teeth for 15 minutes before or after taking a remedy.
- If you have nausea, try *Bryonia*.
- For nausea and vomiting, take *Ipecac*.

Acupressure

- For relief from nausea, firmly press your thumb 2 fingers' width below the crease on your wrist for 1 minute, 2 to 3 times. Repeat on the other wrist. Wrist bands are available that apply pressure to these points.

Point below the wrist

What your doctor would do

Treatment for nausea depends on the cause. If it is due to migraine or infection, then your doctor will prescribe the appropriate drugs. If it is caused by food poisoning, she may advise you to drink plenty of water and to avoid eating anything but very simple food, such as dry toast or crackers, for a day or so until you feel better. Persistent vomiting or vomiting blood will require further investigation to establish the cause.

If you suffer from motion sickness, try sitting where the vehicle is steadiest – in the front seat of the car or bus, as close as possible to the wings of the plane or in the forward or middle cabin of a ship – and looking at the horizon or keeping your eyes closed. Always sit facing the direction of travel. Don't read or do anything that involves looking down for any length of time. Eat little and often before travelling, avoid fatty foods, and drink plenty of liquids, but not orange juice and coffee (which may irritate the stomach).

Your doctor may recommend an over-the-counter medicine to take before travelling.

> **SEE A DOCTOR IF**
>
> - Nausea and vomiting are accompanied by severe abdominal pain, headache, blurred vision or a rash.
> - Vomiting and diarrhoea persist for more than 24 hours.
> - You are taking a new medicine.

> **Warning!**
> Call the doctor if you vomit blood or a dark substance resembling coffee grounds or if your baby cannot keep any milk down.

- For motion sickness, help your balance mechanism by pressing your index finger in the hollow at the back of your jawline. Hold it lightly for 1 minute and breathe deeply. Repeat up to 2 times.

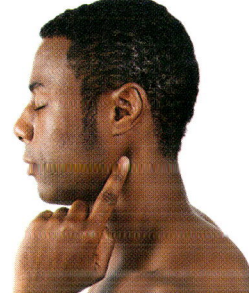

Point for motion sickness just below the ear

STOMACH-ACHE

There are many causes of stomach-ache, including eating spoiled food or food to which you are allergic, and viral infections. Severe abdominal pain may have a more serious cause such as a peptic ulcer or appendicitis.

Your doctor's treatment will depend on the cause. If it is not serious, she may advise you to change your diet or to learn to manage stress. Resting with a covered hot-water bottle on the sore area may ease pain. Acute or persistent pain may require further investigation.

Warning! Call a doctor at once if you have severe or prolonged stomach pain.

Reactions to Food

SYMPTOMS
ALLERGY: ■ Upset stomach with cramps ■ Vomiting and/or diarrhoea ■ Breathing difficulties ■ Swelling of the face, lips, tongue and throat **INTOLERANCE:** ■ Uncomfortably full or bloated feeling ■ Vomiting and/or diarrhoea ■ Flatulence ■ Indigestion and/or heartburn

Many people believe they are allergic to certain foods when, in fact, they have an intolerance. The symptoms are sometimes similar.

Causes
■ A food allergy is a response of the body's immune system to one or more trigger foods – or allergens.
■ If you have a food intolerance, you will feel unwell when you eat a certain food, possibly because your body lacks the enzymes that allow you to digest them.

What your doctor would do
If you think certain foods may upset you, keep a diary of what you eat and how you feel. Your doctor can do tests to help work out which foods don't agree with you. Ask other family members if anyone else has asthma, eczema, hay fever or a food allergy as allergies tend to run in families.

Tablets and drops are available to help people with a milk sugar (lactose) intolerance digest dairy products. Otherwise, the only treatment for food allergy or intolerance is to avoid eating the food that makes you unwell. If you are eating in a restaurant, ask what ingredients are in a dish before you order, and check the ingredients on food labels when shopping.

Alternative Treatments

ACUPRESSURE
To help boost the immune system, place your thumb on the top of your left forearm, 2 thumbs' width from the wrist joint and press firmly. Repeat on the other arm.

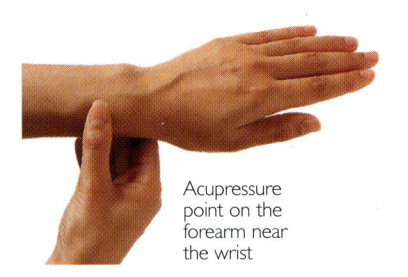

Acupressure point on the forearm near the wrist

ANAPHYLACTIC SHOCK

This is a very serious allergic reaction to a trigger substance such as peanuts, bee stings, shellfish and certain drugs such as aspirin or penicillin. The symptoms include itching and swelling of the mouth, throat and tongue, urticaria all over the body and breathing difficulty. The victim may become unconscious and could die. Treatment is with an adrenaline injection and many people with a serious allergy carry a pre-loaded syringe of adrenaline wherever they go. If you think someone is in anaphylactic shock and unable to help themselves call **999** and give immediate first aid.

FOODS AND SYMPTOMS

FOOD TRIGGERS

DAIRY PRODUCTS Milk, cheese, yogurt, cream, ice cream, cream soups, and certain baked goods and desserts.

EGGS (ESPECIALLY THE WHITES) Eggs are in certain desserts – cakes, ice cream, mousses and sherbets – mayonnaise, salad dressing, waffles and pancakes.

FISH Fresh, canned, smoked or pickled fish, caviar, foods containing fish such as bisques, broths and stews.

SHELLFISH Prawns, mussels, crab, lobster, crayfish, clams, oysters, scallops and seafood dishes.

WHEAT Can be found in cereals, bread products, dry soup mixes and gravies, cakes, pasta, dumplings and products containing flour.

SWEETCORN Some soups and stews, baby foods (with cornflour), baking mixes, processed meats, corn oils, margarine, salad dressings and certain baked goods.

NUTS AND PEANUTS Sweets and baked goods with Brazils, pecans, walnuts, almonds, cashews, hazelnuts, pistachios and peanuts; oils from nuts.

FRUITS Citrus fruits, melons and certain other fruits.

SYMPTOMS

ALLERGY Constipation, diarrhoea and vomiting; occasionally a rash and breathing problems.
INTOLERANCE Bloating, cramping and flatulence.

ALLERGY A rash or intestinal upset. In some susceptible people, eggs cause asthma and eczema.

ALLERGY A rash, red itchy eyes or a runny nose. Can cause asthma, diarrhoea and even anaphylaxis.

ALLERGY Migraine, nausea, intestinal upset, rash, swelling of the skin and anaphylaxis.

ALLERGY Diarrhoea and other intestinal upsets, migraine and eczema.
INTOLERANCE Bloating, cramping, diarrhoea and pale foul-smelling stools. Weight loss or, in a child, failure to thrive.

ALLERGY Rash, breathing problems, diarrhoea and other intestinal upsets; possibly anaphylaxis.

ALLERGY Intestinal upsets and breathing problems; possible anaphylaxis.

ALLERGY Rash on the face, itching or tingling in the mouth.

CALL A DOCTOR IF

- You have violent stomach cramps, vomiting, diarrhoea or continued bloating

CALL A DOCTOR IMMEDIATELY IF:
- Breathing becomes difficult or painful
- Your skin becomes flushed, itchy and develops weals – this could be a sign of anaphylatic shock (see box on opposite page)

Warning!
Never try an elimination diet on your own – it is easier and safer to ask for help from your doctor or a dietitian before you try cutting out any foods you think may be a problem.

Diarrhoea

SYMPTOMS

- Frequent, watery or loose bowel movements over which you have little control
- Abdominal cramps

Diarrhoea is usually a minor complaint and almost everyone experiences it now and again. It normally clears up in a day or two on its own.

Causes
- The most common cause is food poisoning: symptoms tend to appear about six hours after eating.
- Drinking too much coffee can sometimes cause diarrhoea.
- A viral infection of the stomach may be the underlying cause.
- Stress and anxiety may also be to blame.
- Diarrhoea can be a reaction to some types of medicines; check with your doctor if you're taking a new medication.
- A food intolerance or allergy (see pp. 30–31) can cause diarrhoea.
- You may get diarrhoea when on holiday in another country for two reasons: either because you have eaten or drunk contaminated food or water, or simply because the harmless bacteria that normally live in your stomach are not the same as those that you ingest when you are abroad. This can cause your stomach to be upset until it becomes used to the new balance of bacteria. ▶

Alternative treatments

Homeopathy
Arsenicum album is recommended for diarrhoea: take in 6c doses as required. Do not eat, drink or clean your teeth for 15 minutes before or after taking a remedy.

Herbal Remedies
- Infusions of agrimony, plantain or geranium are suggested. To make an infusion, steep a teaspoon of the herb in a cup of hot water for 10 minutes, then strain. You can take 3–4 tablespoons 3 times daily.
- Peppermint or chamomile tea may be soothing as well.

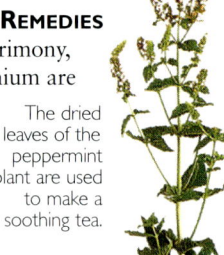

The dried leaves of the peppermint plant are used to make a soothing tea.

Visualization
This can help you deal with the stress that may lead to diarrhoea. Take the phone off the hook. Lie down or sit comfortably and close your eyes. Imagine yourself in a pleasant, peaceful place, such as on a beach, for 15 minutes. Or close your eyes, breathe deeply and listen to soothing music for half an hour.

What your doctor would do

Except in severe cases, diarrhoea does not need medical treatment. To avoid dehydration – when your body loses too much fluid – it is important to replace the fluids and salts in your body which you lose when you have diarrhoea. Children in particular are at risk of dehydration. You can buy suitable "oral rehydration salt" mixtures from a pharmacy or make your own. Dissolve 1 teaspoon of salt and 8 teaspoons of sugar in 1 litre (3½ cups) of water. Measure the quantities carefully. If you have a large enough container you can make bigger quantities at a time, but be sure to keep the proportions accurate. Drink 500 ml (1¾ cups) every hour and eat no solid food until the diarrhoea goes.

Once you feel ready to eat solid foods, start off with bland ones. Doctors often recommend bananas, rice and stewed apple. Drinking the water strained from boiled rice can be helpful, as can eating live yogurt.

Sensible precautions when travelling overseas include drinking only bottled water and avoiding ice cubes in your drinks. Avoid salads, wash and peel fruit carefully and don't eat food that has been kept warm for long.

> **SEE A DOCTOR IF**
>
> - Diarrhoea persists for longer than 48 hours (24 hours in children)
> - There is vomiting
> - There is slimy mucus or blood in the bowel motions.
> - Pale, watery, foul-smelling motions are accompanied by flatulence, stomach cramps and weakness

Acupressure

- Place your fingers on the inside of the leg, about 4 fingers' width above the inner ankle and just behind the shin bone. Massage in an upward movement.
  - Place one fingertip on your abdomen, about 3 fingers' width from your belly button, and massage gently in a circular motion.

Acupressure point above the ankle

Reflexology

The areas said to help the digestive system are on the sole of the foot, just above the heel. Apply pressure to the reflexology point for the small intestine as shown; then work on either side of this point to soothe the large intestine.

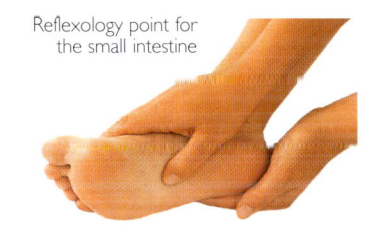

Reflexology point for the small intestine

CONSTIPATION

SYMPTOMS

- Bowel movements occur infrequently – as rarely as once every 3 days in adults, or every 4 days in children
- Bowel movements are difficult and painful
- Stools are hard and compact

Constipation means different things to different people simply because normal bowel movements vary from individual to individual. In general, a person is "regular", or has normal bowel movements, when motions are passed anywhere between as often as three times daily to as infrequently as once every three days. Constipation occurs when there is a change in the normal pattern and when the stools are so hard that it's uncomfortable to pass them.

CAUSES

- The main reason people suffer from constipation is that they don't have enough fibre in their diets. Fibre is found in foods such as fruit and vegetables, wholemeal bread and pasta and brown rice.
- Constipation can also be caused by a lack of fluid.
- Not exercising enough can lead to constipation.
- People suffering from stress may sometimes develop constipation.
- Constipation can be caused by some vitamin supplements, such as iron and calcium, and by certain medicines, such as antihistamines.
- Pregnant women often become constipated.
- If constipation is persistent, it can be a symptom of a more serious disease. ▶

ALTERNATIVE TREATMENTS

HOMEOPATHY
Alumina is recommended if stools are soft but you have to strain to pass them; take 6c every 2 hours for up to 10 doses. Do not eat, drink or clean your teeth for 15 minutes before or after taking a remedy.

HERBAL REMEDIES
An infusion made from dandelion leaves can act as a gentle laxative. Steep 1–2 teaspoons of the dried leaves in a cup of hot water for 10 minutes, then strain. Herbs, such as senna and cascara, can have side-effects and should be used with professional supervision only.

AROMATHERAPY
Mix 3 drops each of the essential oils of rosemary and marjoram and 2 drops of chamomile in 30 ml (6 teaspoons) of almond oil. Gently massage in a clockwise direction around the belly button.

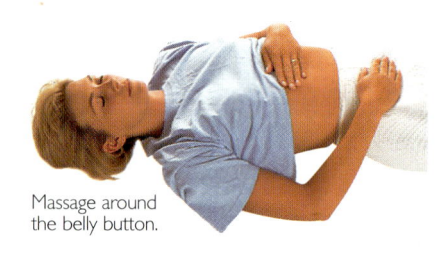

Massage around the belly button.

What your doctor would do
Your doctor will ask you some routine questions to rule out any serious cause for constipation – for example, you may be asked whether there is any blood in your motions. You will then be given advice about your diet and lifestyle.

In some cases, the doctor may recommend one of several types of laxative, such as one containing lactulose – a type of sugar – which will help the motions pass more easily. You should avoid over-the-counter laxatives, except for those that contain fibre or other bulking ingredients. If used too often, they can make the bowels "lazy" or hide a serious problem. It is much healthier to follow these self-help measures:

- Eat at least five portions of fresh fruit, salad and vegetables every day.
- Switch to wholemeal bread, and eat plenty of pulses, brown rice and wholemeal pasta.
- Many people don't drink nearly enough fluid. Try to drink at least eight glasses of water or other fluid a day.
- Try to take some form of brisk exercise at least five times a week for half an hour.

SEE A DOCTOR IF
- Constipation persists for longer than a week
- There is blood in your stools, or you have severe, prolonged or repeated abdominal pain, or a fever
- Constipation starts shortly after you have begun new medication

Reflexology
Work on the pressure point said to relate to the intestines. Gently apply pressure to the centre of the foot, above the heel; then massage for 10 minutes.

Acupressure
- Press a fingertip on the back of the arm, 4 fingers' width from the wrist. Massage in a circular motion.

Acupressure point on the back of forearm

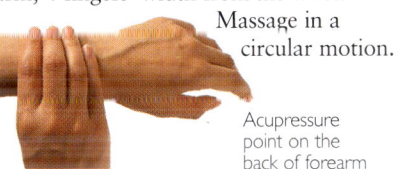

- Bend your arm, placing your hand on the opposite shoulder. Press the thumb of your other hand deeply into the outer edge of the elbow crease in the bent arm and hold for 1 minute. Repeat on the other arm.

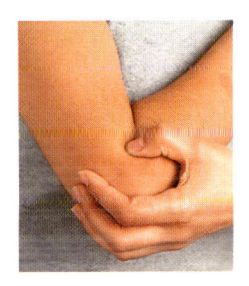

Acupressure point at the elbow

Haemorrhoids

SYMPTOMS

- Soreness and itching of the anal area
- A feeling of "fullness" around the area
- Bleeding from the anus
- Constipation
- A lump or swelling by the anus
- A discharge of mucus from the anus

Also known as piles, haemorrhoids are swollen veins that occur in the lining of the rectum and anus. Internal haemorrhoids develop in the rectum: normally, they can't be seen or felt and the only symptom may be bleeding. Sometimes, however, they can prolapse, or fall down, into the anus, causing pain.

External haemorrhoids develop in the anus and are painful. These, too, may prolapse and protrude out of the anus. This type of prolapsed haemorrhoid can develop a blood clot, which may look serious and be painful, but should disappear on its own in about a week.

Causes
- Haemorrhoids often develop in people who are constipated (see pp. 34–35) because straining to pass motions puts pressure on the veins in the rectum and anus. Hard motions also irritate the veins.
- Pregnancy and childbirth can encourage haemorrhoids.
- People who stand or sit for long periods are more likely to develop haemorrhoids.
- Obesity can also be a trigger. ▶

Alternative treatments

Homeopathy
A homeopath may suggest the remedies below at 12x dosages (do not eat, drink or clean your teeth for 15 minutes before or after taking one):
- *Hamamelis* for a sore, bleeding anus.
- *Aesculus* for sharp rectum pain that worsens when passing motions.
- *Sulphur* to reduce itching and burning.

Hamamelis virginiana, witch hazel, the source for *Hamamelis*

Herbal Remedies
- Try an ointment made from pilewort: simmer 2 tablespoons of the herb in 200 g (7 ounces) of petroleum jelly for 10 minutes. Cool before use.
- To reduce itching and pain, dab witch hazel on the area.
- You can use an infusion of yarrow (steep 1–2 teaspoons of the dried herb in a cup of hot water for 10 minutes) as a compress: dip a clean cloth or towel into the warm infusion and apply to the affected area until the cloth is cold.

Pilewort can be used in an ointment.

What your doctor would do

To prevent haemorrhoids degenerating from a minor discomfort and embarrassment to something more serious, it is important to take action as soon as you suspect you may have them. Your doctor will need to examine the area, possibly by inserting a special tube with a light on the end, to rule out the possibility of other more serious condtions.

Mild cases can be controlled by diet, so your doctor may suggest ways of including more fibre-rich foods. You may also be given a corticosteroid cream or suppositories that will help reduce the swelling. Larger haemorrhoids may be removed in a simple and painless procedure requiring no anaesthetic; prolapsed haemorrhoids may need surgery under anaesthetic.

These are steps that you can take to help prevent haemorrhoids:
- Increase your intake of fibre: make sure you have five portions of fresh fruits and vegetables every day, and try to eat more pulses, wholemeal bread and pasta and brown rice.
- Try to drink at least eight glasses of water a day.
- Exercise at least twice a week for half an hour. This can help prevent constipation, which can cause haemorrhoids.

SEE A DOCTOR IF

- You have anal bleeding and never had haemorrhoids before
- If you have chronic anal bleeding – either daily or weekly – even if you have already been diagnosed as having haemorrhoids

Aromatherapy

- Cypress, juniper, peppermint and chamomile oils are recommended: mix a few drops of each of these essential oils into a carrier oil, such as almond or soya bean, and apply to the affected area.
- Cypress, juniper, peppermint and chamomile oils can also be used in a warm bath. Pour a few drops directly into the water.
- To relieve the constipation that can cause and irritate haemorrhoids, massage the stomach area with a mixture of 3 drops each of the essential oils of rosemary and marjoram and 2 drops of chamomile in 30 ml (6 teaspoons) of almond oil. Gently massage in a clockwise direction around the navel, alternately applying and releasing pressure. **Warning!** Do not use juniper oil if pregnant.

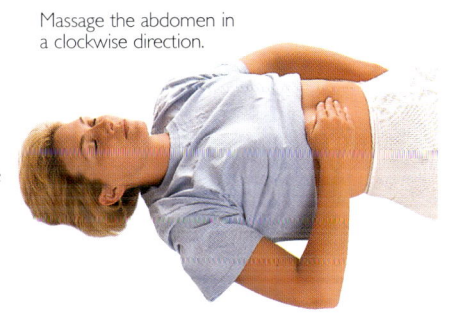

Massage the abdomen in a clockwise direction.

IRRITABLE BOWEL SYNDROME

SYMPTOMS

- Abdominal cramps
- Bloating
- Diarrhoea or constipation
- Intestinal wind

Also known as spastic colon or irritable colon, irritable bowel syndrome (IBS) is a condition in which some of the muscles in the colon fail to move as they should – in synchronized contractions – and go into spasm instead. It is one of the most common digestive problems, affecting up to 20 percent of adults. It occurs more frequently in women than in men and usually starts in early adulthood.

The symptoms of irritable bowel syndrome are sometimes – but not always – relieved by passing wind or a bowel motion but the sufferer may be left with the feeling that he or she has been unable to empty the bowels properly. It is common for symptoms to subside or disappear for some time, but attacks usually recur frequently.

CAUSES
No one knows for sure what causes IBS; the intestines are otherwise normal and there's no unexplained weight loss.
- Stress is believed to be one important cause of IBS.
- An intolerance to certain foods may be another factor (see pp. 30–31). ▶

ALTERNATIVE TREATMENTS

HOMEOPATHY
Do not eat, drink or brush your teeth for 15 minutes before or after taking a remedy.
- *Argentum nitricum* 6x, *Nux vomica* 30x, and *Ignatia* 6c are recommended for various bowel ailments, ranging from diarrhoea to constipation or bowel spasms. Follow instructions on the label.

HERBAL REMEDIES
Peppermint can help relax the intestines. You can make an infusion by steeping 1 teaspoon of the dried herb in a cup of boiling water for 30 minutes. Strain and drink 3 cups a day.

VISUALIZATION
To cope better with stress, close your eyes and for 15 minutes imagine yourself in a pleasant, peaceful place,

Lie down, relax your muscles and visualize a quiet place.

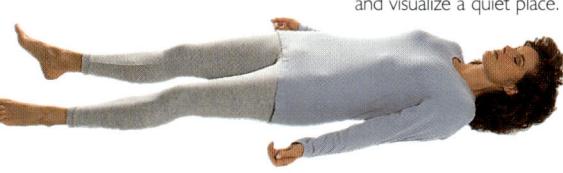

What your doctor would do

There is no test for irritable bowel syndrome, but your doctor will want to rule out other more serious conditions. She will examine you and may want to look inside your anus with a special light. Swabs may be taken, or you may be asked to bring in a stool sample.

There's no cure for irritable bowel syndrome, but your doctor can make suggestions of how you can try to reduce the symptoms:

- After discussing your diet, the doctor may suggest you eat less fat and more fibre. Make sure you have five portions of fresh fruits and vegetables every day, and eat plenty of pulses, wholemeal bread and pasta and brown rice.
- Your doctor may ask you about your emotional state and how you deal with stress. She may recommend several ways to reduce stress.
- In severe cases, your doctor may prescribe drugs that can reduce the spasms.

SEE A DOCTOR IF

- You have pain in the lower left abdomen, accompanied by a fever
- There is blood in your motions
- You have a fever and unexplained weight loss
- There is a change in the frequency of your motions
- Mucus is present

---

such as on a deserted beach. Lying down helps, but you can also do this in a sitting position.

Reflexology

- The reflexology point for your intestines is above the heel of the foot. To ease the symptoms of IBS, first apply pressure to the point, then massage the area for 10 minutes.
- To reduce stress, massage the solar

Massaging this point reduces intestinal upsets.

Massage this point to reduce stress.

plexus point near the inside edge at the bottom of the ball of the big toe.

Acupressure

To reduce pain, press your index fingers 2 fingers' widths' away from each side of your navel for 1 minute and release; repeat 5 times.

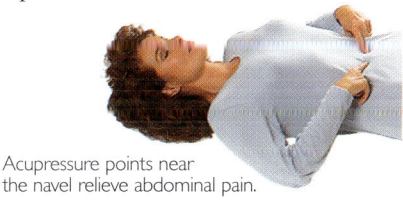

Acupressure points near the navel relieve abdominal pain.

Food Poisoning

SYMPTOMS

- Abdominal pain
- Vomiting
- Diarrhoea

CALL A DOCTOR IF

- You have repeated bouts of vomiting
- Diarrhoea is severe or lasts over 48 hours for an adult, 24 for a child

Warning!
Call a doctor immediately if a person with food poisoning collapses.

This is a general name for any illness that results from eating spoiled food. The symptoms may be mild and last only a day or so, but in extreme cases they may be life-threatening.

Causes
- Eating food that has been contaminated with bacteria, viruses or poisons from them. Often everyone who ate the bad food becomes ill.
- One form of food poisoning is caused by *Salmonella* bacteria, which may be present in undercooked poultry, undercooked eggs or foods made with raw eggs.

The *E. coli* bacteria which are sometimes found in raw or undercooked meat – particularly minced meat – can cause a severe form of food poisoning.

What your doctor would do
Most food poisoning goes away after a few days and does not require medical treatment. You should avoid solid food for at least 24 hours and drink plenty of fluids.

If the vomiting and diarrhoea are severe, the doctor may send samples to be analysed. In severe cases, it may be necessary for the stomach to be washed out in hospital, but most medical treatment concentrates on replacing lost fluids.

Alternative Treatments

Herbal Remedies
Ginger tea relieves nausea. Drink a cup every 2 hours; or take 2 ginger capsules.

Homeopathy
You can take 12c of *Arsenicum album* or *Nux vomica* every 3 hours. Do not eat, drink or brush your teeth for 15 minutes before or after taking a remedy.

Acupressure
For nausea, apply pressure with your thumb on your inner forearm, 2 fingers' width below the wrist crease for 1 minute.

AVOIDING FOOD POISONING

- Always wash your hands before handling food.
- Be careful when cutting meat: make sure you wash the place where it was cut and the knife you used before bringing them into contact with other food. Wash your hands after touching raw meat. Don't let juices from raw meat drip on to other food in the refrigerator.
- Make sure frozen poultry is thawed completely and thoroughly cooked.
- Never eat: mussels that do not open when boiled; food from cans that are bulging; food that smells or tastes bad.

ACHES & PAINS

Everyone, at some stage, experiences aches and pains, which may range from muscle cramp to back pain or gout. The musculoskeletal system consists of bones, muscles, ligaments, tendons and joints, all of which can cause pain if they are not working in harmony.

Some of these conditions, for example sprains, strains and torn ligaments, may result from sudden exertion, from not warming up sufficiently before exercise, or from playing sports such as football. Others affect the joints and include gout, rheumatoid arthritis and osteoarthritis.

This section outlines a variety of ways of alleviating aches and pains, including rest, a change in diet, over-the-counter painkillers, and alternative therapies; some, however, may need surgery.

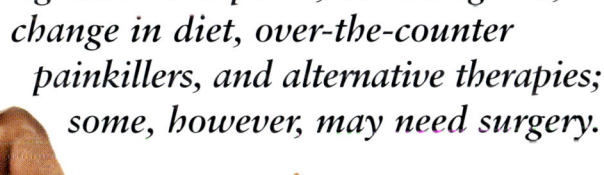

Strains & Sprains

SYMPTOMS

Strains:
- Pain
- Swelling
- Bruising

Sprains:
- Pain
- Some stiffness
- Immediate swelling

Torn knee or ankle ligaments:
- Considerable pain
- The knee or ankle looks a strange shape
- You are unable to put any weight on the leg

Tendinitis:
- Pain or tenderness
- Restricted movement of the muscle

Causes
- A strained muscle may result from sudden strenuous exertion or not warming up properly before exercise. Fibres are stretched or even torn, leading to bleeding in the damaged area.
- A sprain usually happens after a sudden, abnormal movement in that part of the body.
- Torn ligaments in the knee or ankle are a hazard of football and similar sports – a sudden twist of the joint while your weight is on that leg can do considerable damage.
- Tendinitis results from repeated stressful movements performed at work or when playing sports.

What your doctor would do
For strains and sprains, doctors recommend RICE: rest, ice (applied to the area to reduce internal bleeding and swelling), compression (a carefully applied elastic bandage) and elevation (raise the part up to help prevent swelling). You may need anti-inflammatory painkillers.

Torn ligaments may need surgical repair, or a plaster cast to keep the joint immobile. Tendinitis generally responds to avoidance of the movement which caused it, or to improved positioning and frequent stretching during the movement as well as – in the short-term – anti-inflammatory drugs. ▶

Alternative treatments

Aromatherapy
- For sprains, add 2 drops each of the essential oils of hyssop and sweet marjoram to a warm bath.
- Alternatively, massage the affected area with 2 drops each of hyssop and sweet marjoram oils mixed with a teaspoon of a carrier oil such as almond. Then apply a cold compress: add 5 drops of each of the essential oils to just enough water to soak a handkerchief or face cloth. You can wrap cling film around the compress to hold it in place. **Warning!** Do not use hyssop oil if pregnant.

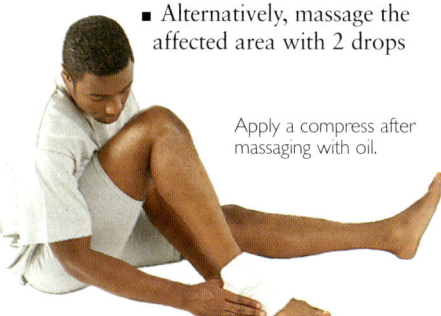

Apply a compress after massaging with oil.

Homeopathy
Do not eat, drink or clean your teeth for 15 minutes before or after taking a remedy.
- For muscle strains, take *Arnica* 30c

Rotator cuff tendinitis (at back of shoulder) due to overhead motions, such as serving in tennis.

Tennis elbow due to repetitive motions.

Hamstring strain is common in runners.

Shin pain occurs when overuse makes the muscles tear and is common in joggers.

A sprained ankle occurs when the ligaments – the bands of tissue connecting the bones – are damaged.

Shoulder joint dislocation: the bones pull apart, stretching the tissues holding them in place.

Lumbar, or lower back, strain happens when the fibres of the muscles are pulled too far apart.

Pain in the knee as a result of injury may be caused by torn ligament or cartilage – the tissue that lines joints and prevents friction between bones.

Achilles tendinitis (at the back of the ankle) occurs when the tendon – the strong tissue that joins the calf muscle to the heel-bone – is inflamed.

SEE A DOCTOR IF

- You can't use the affected muscle or joint, or it's very painful
- The problem joint, such as the knee, ankle or wrist, looks the wrong shape
- You think the affected area may have a ligament or muscle tear
- You suspect a bone may be broken

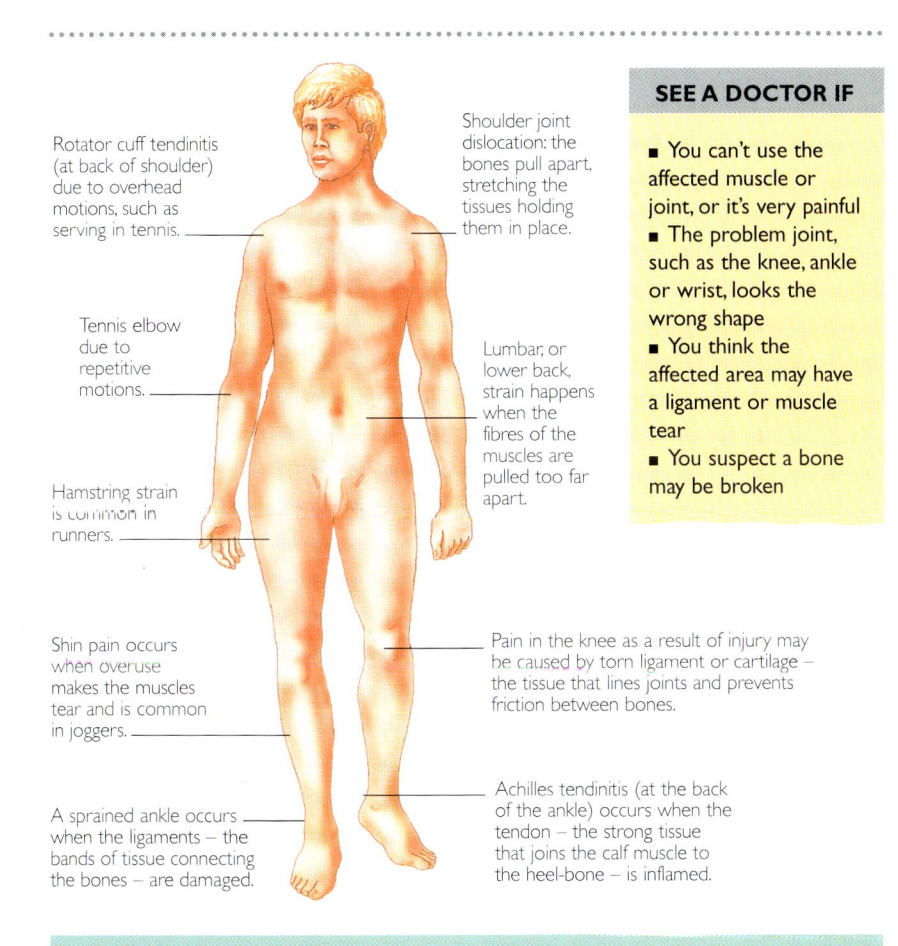

every half hour, for 10 doses. Then take *Rhus toxicodendron* 6c 4 times a day until the pain disappears.

■ If you have a sprain or tendinitis, try *Arnica* 30c every half hour, for 10 doses, and follow with *Ruta* 6c 4 times a day until the pain subsides.

Herbal Remedies

Comfrey helps to reduce swelling and bruising from sprains and strains. Make a

Use dried comfrey to reduce swelling.

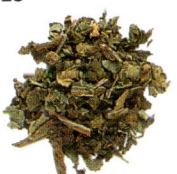

compress by dipping a clean cloth in a cold comfrey infusion and applying to the affected area. (To make an infusion, steep 1–2 teaspoons of dried comfrey in a cup of hot water for about 10 minutes; then strain and cool.) Or, rub in some comfrey cream.

Acupressure

Apply gentle pressure approximately 15 cm (6 inches) away from the injury, not on the injury itself. For knee problems, find the pressure point on the outside of the leg, 4 fingers' width below the kneecap.

BURSITIS

SYMPTOMS

- Inflammation, swelling and pain in a shoulder, elbow, hip or knee following prolonged use of that joint
- Difficulty in moving the joint, with or without pain

SEE A DOCTOR IF

- Symptoms persist for more than a few days
- Anti-inflammatory drugs or painkillers fail to reduce the swelling

CAUSES

Bursitis is inflammation of a bursa, a fluid-filled pad that acts as a cushion where tendons or muscles cross bones. It happens when repeated pressure is put on a joint such as a knee, elbow, shoulder or hip. It often occurs in people who participate in sports or manual labour.

WHAT YOUR DOCTOR WOULD DO

Rest the area as much as you can; the inflammation should go away of its own accord within about 10 days. Applying ice-cold compresses to the area and taking over-the-counter anti-inflammatory painkillers will help with swelling and pain. In severe cases he may need to inject anti-inflammatory drugs. Physiotherapy can also help.

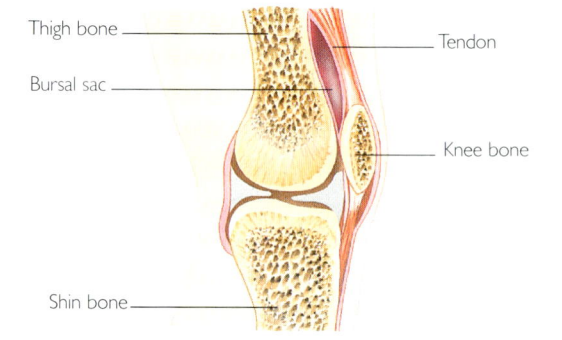

Thigh bone
Tendon
Bursal sac
Knee bone
Shin bone

ALTERNATIVE TREATMENTS

HERBAL REMEDIES
To ease pain, rub a tincture of lobelia and cramp bark on the affected area. To make a tincture, half-fill a screw-topped jar with the chopped or ground herbs, fill the jar with alcohol (vodka is ideal) and store in a warm dark place. Shake twice daily. After 2 weeks, decant into another jar and store in a cool place.

HOMEOPATHY
Take *Apis* 6x every 2 hours for swelling and pain. Do not eat, drink or clean your teeth for 15 minutes before or after taking a remedy.

PREVENTING BURSITIS

- Always remember to warm up and cool down properly before and after doing any form of exercise. This will help to avoid putting strain on your joints.
- When doing activities that require being on your knees, such as gardening, wear kneepads or use a foam rubber mat to help ease the pressure on the kneecaps.
- If you have a problem with a particular joint, wear a crepe or tubular elastic bandage to support it.

Repetitive Strain Injury

Symptoms

- Pain, weakness, swelling and burning in the affected area

See a doctor if

- Pain is accompanied by stiffness in the hands or fingers and/or swollen joints
- Pain in your wrist or hand occurs after a fall or other accident
- Pain becomes worse at night
- Your fingers and hands turn white and then red in cold weather

Also known as RSI and work-related upper limb disorder, repetitive strain injury is a disorder that usually affects the hand, thumb, neck, elbow and shoulder. Usually the sheath that surrounds a tendon (which attaches a muscle to a bone) becomes inflamed.

Causes

- It is caused by overuse of the affected area and by poor posture and is common in people who spend many hours at a computer keyboard, play a lot of sport or do any repetitive physical work. Other examples include tennis elbow and writer's cramp.

What your doctor would do

Short-term treatments for RSI include rest, cold compresses and anti-inflammatory painkillers. For example, for RSI of the hand and wrist, you may need to wear a splint and change your working practices. Make sure your chair is comfortable and pay attention to your posture. If you work at a computer, take a 10-minute break from the screen every hour. Your elbows should not rest below your wrists. In the most severe cases of RSI, sufferers have found themselves unable to continue in their occupation, so take advice about preventive measures as soon as you notice any problem.

Alternative treatments

Herbal Remedies

Try a hot poultice made from comfrey, slippery elm, linseed or marshmallow:
- Boil the fresh leaves of your chosen herb and when cool enough to handle, squeeze out any extra liquid. Apply the herbs directly to the affected area using a piece of gauze to keep the leaves in place.
- You can use the dried herb by adding hot water to make a paste and holding it in place with gauze.

Comfrey
Slippery elm
Marshmallow
Linseed

Homeopathy

- To relieve pain, rub *Arnica* cream into the affected area.
- Take *Arnica* 6x or *Aconite* 6x twice a day for 3 days. Do not eat, drink or clean your teeth 15 minutes before or after taking a remedy.

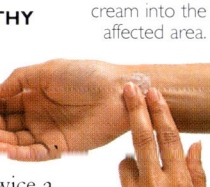

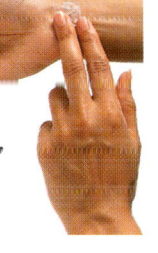

Rub *Arnica* cream into the affected area.

Muscle Cramp

SYMPTOMS

- Sudden stabbing pain which usually passes after a short while

RESTLESS LEGS

This is the name given to an uncomfortable syndrome in which the legs ache, feel hot and uncomfortable and need to keep moving around. It often occurs at night, can run in families and may be linked to smoking and caffeine consumption.
If it is severe, your doctor may prescribe drugs. Otherwise, if you smoke or drink a lot of coffee or cola, cut down or stop.

A cramp happens when muscles contract very tightly and don't release again as they should do – sometimes because the various chemicals in the muscles are out of balance. The muscle goes into a painful spasm and feels solid to the touch.

Causes

- A cramp often happens during or after exercise, which can cause a build-up of certain chemicals in the body.
- Excessive sweating can lead to a cramp because of a chemical imbalance.
- A cramp can occur in the middle of the night. No one really knows what causes this, although poor circulation may be one explanation (this is different from restless legs; see box, left).

What your doctor would do

There isn't a cure for cramp. The best treatment is to massage the muscle that hurts, warm it and stretch it gently. To help prevent cramp, make sure you drink plenty of fluid (at least eight glasses a day), particularly in hot weather. To prevent night cramp, try doing stretching exercises after a warm bath before going to bed.

Alternative treatments

Herbal Remedies
An infusion of ginkgo can help ease cramp. Steep 2 teaspoons of the dried herb in a cup of boiling water for 15 minutes and strain. Drink 3 cups a day.

Acupressure
For cramp in the calf, press on the area at the lower end of the calf muscle, where it bulges, for 2–3 minutes.

Aromatherapy
Massage the affected muscle with a few drops each of the essential oils of basil and marjoram, diluted in 2½ teaspoons of warmed almond oil.
Warning! Do not use marjoram or basil essential oils if pregnant.

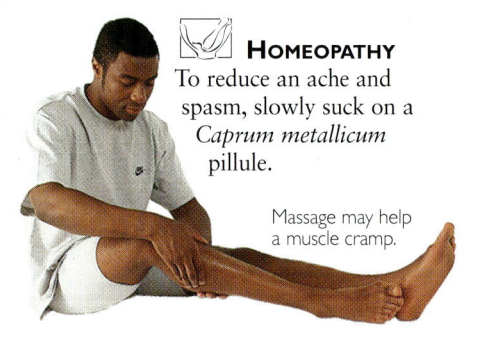

Homeopathy
To reduce an ache and spasm, slowly suck on a *Caprum metallicum* pillule.

Massage may help a muscle cramp.

Neck & Shoulder Pain

Symptoms

- A dull pain and difficulty in moving your head or shoulder

Whiplash:
- Sudden pain in the neck following an injury

See a Doctor If

- Neck pain occurs after an accident
- Neck pain persists for longer than 1 day
- A stiff neck is accompanied by fever, severe headache and vomiting – these could be symptoms of meningitis

Neck and shoulder pain and stiffness is very common; it is often referred to as fibrositis, a term simply meaning inflammation of fibrous tissue. A whiplash injury of the neck results from damage to the soft tissue, ligaments and joints.

Causes
- Sleeping awkwardly, injury, and muscle tension from stress can cause pain and stiffness in the area.
- A sudden jerking of the neck can cause whiplash; this commonly occurs in a car accident.

What Your Doctor Would Do
For stiffness and pain in the neck and shoulder, use hot or cold compresses or packs and take over-the-counter anti-inflammatory painkillers. If it is no better within 24 hours, see your doctor, who may recommend certain exercises. The doctor may need to rule out a more serious condition.

If you think you have a whiplash injury, apply ice to the painful area and see your doctor right away. Your doctor may want to immobilize your neck in an orthopaedic collar for up to a week.

Alternative Treatments

Acupressure
- For neck pain, apply pressure with the tips of your index fingers pressing upward toward your head. There are 2 points between the bottom of the skull and the top of the neck muscles, each 2 fingers' width from the centre of the vertebrae running down your neck.
- To relieve shoulder pain, press the point on the muscle midway between the point of your shoulder and your neck for up to 3 minutes.

Acupressure points for neck pain (left) and shoulder pain (right)

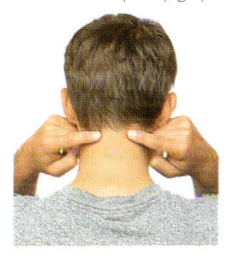

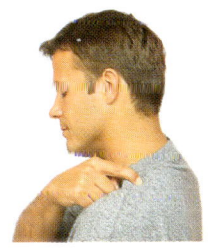

Aromatherapy
Add a few drops of the essential oil of rosemary to bath water. Or mix the drops in 2½ teaspoons of a carrier oil, such as almond or soya bean; massage it into the painful area.

Back Pain

Symptoms

Lumbago:
- Pain in the lower back after strenuous activity or heavy lifting
- An ache in the lower or middle back after sitting or standing for long periods

Fibrositis:
- Pain and tenderness in larger back muscles

Sciatica:
- Pain in the buttock and down the thigh, sometimes as far as the foot

Disc pain:
- Lower back pain, sometimes with sciatica
- Numbness and tingling

Causes
- **Lumbago** is usually caused by poor posture and sitting incorrectly; overexertion, careless lifting; the weight and the ligament relaxation of pregnancy; lack of sleep; stress.
- **Fibrositis** is the name sometimes given to muscle pain and stiffness and is often caused by tension and poor posture.
- **Sciatica** results from pressure on the sciatic nerve, usually from a tense muscle or a slipped disc.
- **Disc pain** may result from a slipped disc after sudden strenuous and awkward activity, but is more usually caused by wear and tear to the discs.

What your doctor would do
Your doctor will examine you, rule out a urine infection and, if necessary, arrange an X-ray or scan.

For most back pain, the doctor will recommend anti-inflammatory painkillers, heat and, perhaps, massage, careful stretching exercises and other physiotherapy. Rest is no longer recommended for most back pain. However, a slipped disc requires several weeks of bed rest. ▶

Alternative treatments

Homeopathy
Take 6c of any of the following remedies 4 times a day for up to 2 weeks. Do not eat, drink or clean your teeth for 15 minutes before or after taking a remedy.
- *Bryonia* is suggested for sharp pain.
- Try *Nux vomica* for persistent pain.
- *Arnica* is good for sore muscles.
- *Rhus toxicodendron* is useful for sharp pain and for easing stiffness in the morning.

Acupressure
- For lower back pain, follow a line from the point between your little and ring fingers to just below your wrist and apply pressure for 3 minutes.
- Also for lower back pain, press with both thumbs on either side of the spine just above the pelvis for 1 minute, then gently massage.

Acupressure point for lower back pain

Herbal Remedies
To make an infusion for one of the following teas, steep a tea bag or a teaspoon of the dried herb in a cup of

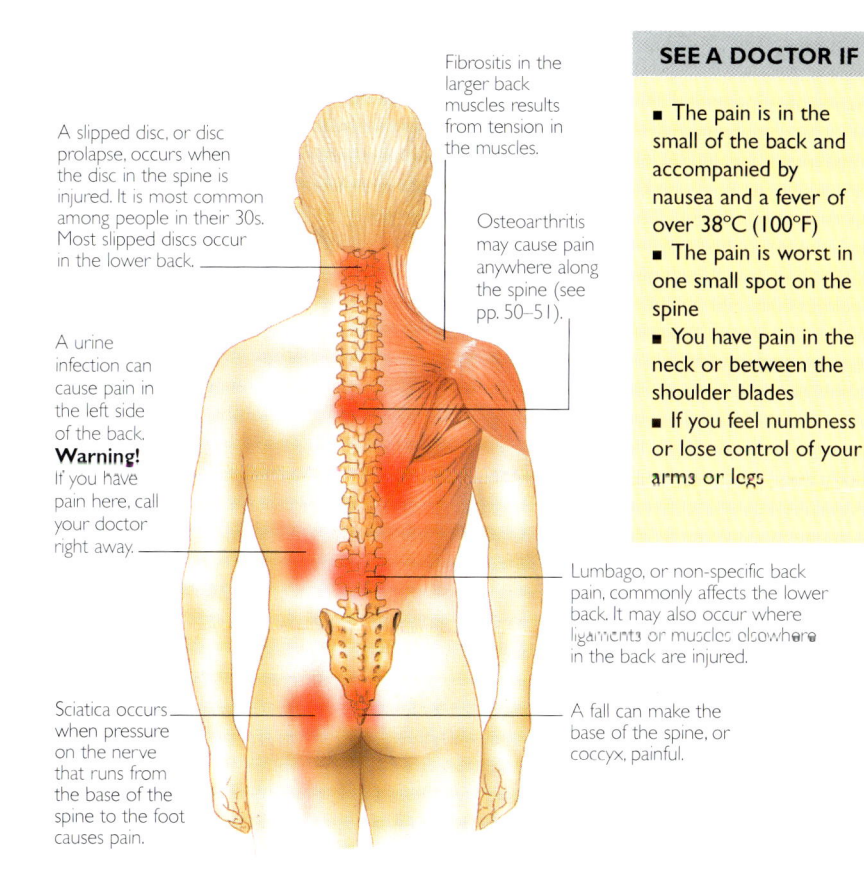

A slipped disc, or disc prolapse, occurs when the disc in the spine is injured. It is most common among people in their 30s. Most slipped discs occur in the lower back.

Fibrositis in the larger back muscles results from tension in the muscles.

Osteoarthritis may cause pain anywhere along the spine (see pp. 50–51).

A urine infection can cause pain in the left side of the back.
Warning! If you have pain here, call your doctor right away.

Lumbago, or non-specific back pain, commonly affects the lower back. It may also occur where ligaments or muscles elsewhere in the back are injured.

Sciatica occurs when pressure on the nerve that runs from the base of the spine to the foot causes pain.

A fall can make the base of the spine, or coccyx, painful.

SEE A DOCTOR IF

- The pain is in the small of the back and accompanied by nausea and a fever of over 38°C (100°F)
- The pain is worst in one small spot on the spine
- You have pain in the neck or between the shoulder blades
- If you feel numbness or lose control of your arms or legs

3

---

boiling water for 5 minutes. Strain if necessary and add honey if you like.
- Try white willow for reducing pain.
- Lobelia will help reduce inflammation.
- For sciatica, try white willow, black cohosh, skullcap or rosemary.

AROMATHERAPY

A few drops of the essential oils of rosemary, chamomile or lavender can be added to bath water. Or mix the drops in 2½ teaspoons of a carrier oil, such as almond or soya bean, and massage it into the affected area. In addition, try geranium oil for sciatica.

REFLEXOLOGY

For 1 minute, gently apply pressure to one of the reflexology points.

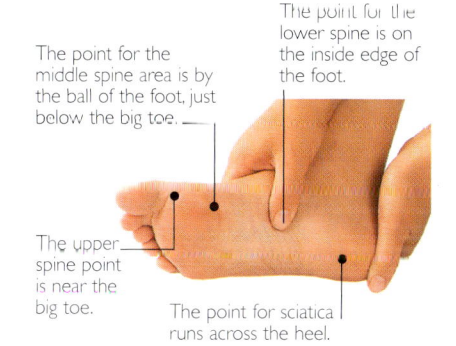

The point for the middle spine area is by the ball of the foot, just below the big toe.

The point for the lower spine is on the inside edge of the foot.

The upper spine point is near the big toe.

The point for sciatica runs across the heel.

Osteoarthritis

SYMPTOMS

- Pain and stiffness in a joint or joints without obvious swelling, particularly in the hip, knees, spine and hands
- Eventually, difficulty in moving the joints
- In a few cases, muscle inflammation
- Occasionally, extreme pain from muscle or nerve damage caused by bone spurs

Causes

- Doctors don't know exactly what causes osteoarthritis, although it affects more women than men and sometimes runs in some families. It can follow an injury to a joint. It is also generally thought to be part of getting older.
- If osteoarthritis causes joints to become deformed, they can develop bone spurs, an abnormal bony growth, which can press on surrounding muscles and nerves. ▶

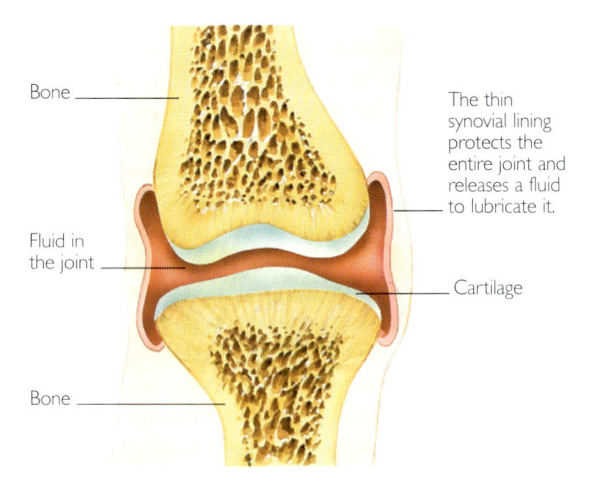

In a healthy joint, cartilage – a tough smooth tissue – covers the ends of bones where two of them meet, acting as a cushion.

Bone

Fluid in the joint

Bone

The thin synovial lining protects the entire joint and releases a fluid to lubricate it.

Cartilage

Alternative treatments

Homeopathy

Take 6c of one of these remedies 4 times daily, for up to 2 weeks. Do not eat, drink or clean your teeth for 15 minutes beforehand or afterward.
- *Rhus toxicodendron* is recommended for pain with stiffness brought on by dampness and rest.
- *Bryonia* is suggested for severe pain with movement.

Bryonia

Herbal Remedies

These are just a few of the remedies that a herbalist may suggest to help relieve the symptoms of osteoarthritis. To make a tincture, half-fill a large screw-topped jar with the herb, fill the jar with alcohol (vodka is ideal) and store in a warm place away from the sun. Shake the jar twice a day. After 2 weeks, decant the mixture into another jar and store in a cool place.

Devil's claw can be used to make a tincture.

What your doctor would do

Your doctor may take X-rays to examine the bones for osteoarthritis. There is no cure, but treatments are aimed at reducing the pain and discomfort. They include anti-inflammatory painkillers and perhaps injections into the affected joints. Applying heat to the affected area may be recommended. Gentle, regular exercise is a good idea as it keeps the muscles either side of the affected joint in good condition, and physiotherapy may be suggested too.

See a doctor if

- You notice that your arms, legs or back develop pain and stiffness after sitting for short periods or sleeping overnight.

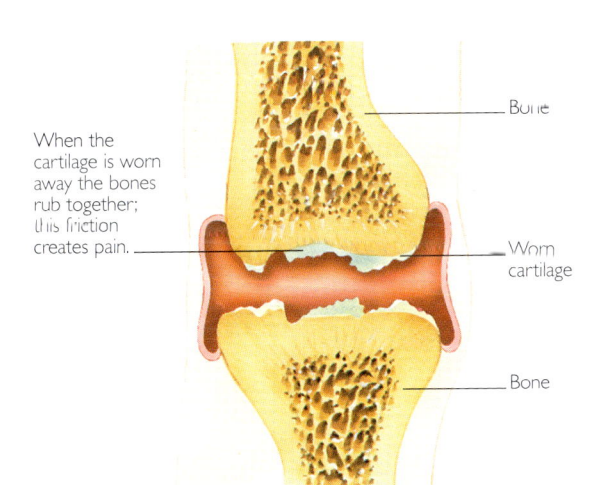

When the cartilage is worn away the bones rub together; this friction creates pain.

Bone

Worn cartilage

Bone

In osteoarthritis, the most common type of arthritis, the cartilage in the joint wears away after years of use. This is sometimes referred to as wear-and-tear arthritis.

- Take 1 tablespoon of a tincture made from devil's claw daily.
- For relief from pain, try 1 teaspoon 3 times daily of a tincture of 2 parts willow and 1 part each of nettle and black cohosh.
- To ease muscle tension, you can rub the affected area with a tincture of lobelia and cramp bark.

Aromatherapy
Gently massage the affected area with a few drops of tiger balm, chamomile or lavender essential oil in 2½ teaspoons of a carrier oil such as almond or soya bean.

Reflexology
To relieve pain in the hip or knee joint, gently apply pressure for 1 minute to the relevant reflexology point shown below. Use the right foot for joints on the right side of the body, the left foot for those on the left side. **Warning!** Do not do this if you are pregnant.

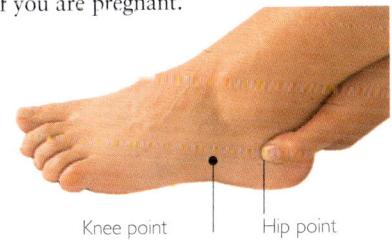

Knee point | Hip point

Rheumatoid Arthritis

SYMPTOMS

- Pain, swelling and stiffness in the arms, legs, wrists or fingers on both sides of the body
- Fatigue
- Symptoms are more severe on awakening
- In children, loss of appetite, fever, rash on the arms and legs

SEE A DOCTOR IF

- Joints suddenly become swollen, stiff and painful.
- A rash appears on a child's armpits, wrists, knees or ankles along with a fever and loss of appetite

Causes
This condition is more common in women and often begins after 40, but can happen at any time. It is thought to be caused by a virus or other trigger making the immune system attack the body's own tissues.

What your doctor would do
Your doctor may prescribe anti-inflammatory drugs. Rest, heat compresses and gentle exercise may be recommended. Physiotherapy can help relieve pain and give greater mobility in the affected area. In extreme cases, surgery may be necessary to replace joints with artificial ones.

In rheumatoid arthritis, the synovial lining becomes inflamed and causes the cartilage to break down. (See p. 50 for a healthy joint.)

The sinovial lining thickens and becomes inflamed.

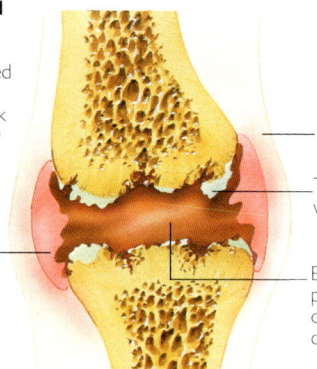

The joint looks swollen and misshapen.

The cartilage wears away.

Extra fluid puts pressure on the cartilage.

Alternative Treatments

Herbal Remedies
To relieve the pain, try a tincture of willow bark. To prepare a tincture, half-fill a large screw-topped jar with the herb, fill the jar up with alcohol (vodka is ideal) and store in a warm dark place. Shake the jar twice a day. After 2 weeks, decant into another jar and store in a cool place. Take 1 teaspoon 3 times daily.

Homeopathy
Take 6c of *Bryonia* 4 times daily, up to 2 weeks. For 15 minutes before or after taking a remedy, do not eat, drink or clean your teeth.

Aromatherapy
Gently massage the joints with tiger balm, or use a few drops of chamomile or lavender essential oil diluted in a carrier oil such as almond or soya bean.

Massage the oils into the affected joint.

Gout

SYMPTOMS

- Sudden, unexpected sharp pain in the joint of a big toe, ankle, finger or knee that lasts no more than a week and may recur
- Swelling and inflammation in the affected joint, as well as a sensation of heat
- In an extreme case, fever and chills

SEE A DOCTOR IF

- If severe pain lasts more than 3 days or recurs, or if it occurs with fever and chills
- The symptoms increase while taking medicine prescribed by your doctor

Gout is a form of arthritis that mainly affects such joints as the big toe, knees, fingers and elbows. It occurs when an extremely high level of uric acid in the blood causes crystals to be deposited in a joint. Gout is most common in middle-aged men.

Causes

- Men who are overweight or taking diuretics for high blood pressure are prone to gout.
- Heredity is a factor in half of the cases.
- An injury, surgery, stress and reactions to alcohol and certain drugs, such as aspirin and antibiotics, can cause gout.
- Kidney disorders and certain enzyme deficiencies can lead to gout.
- Certain foods can trigger gout.

What your doctor would do

Your doctor will probably suggest taking painkillers or an anti-inflammatory drug. Drugs may also be given to help prevent the build-up of crystals but it is possible to control this by what you eat. If you have gout, avoid eating offal, shellfish, processed meat and fish (especially sardines), tinned fish, asparagus, spinach, most types of dried beans, chocolate, beer and red wine.

Alternative Treatments

Homeopathy

You can take 6x doses of *Arnica*, *Colchicum* or *Belladonna* every 2 hours for up to 12 doses. Do not eat, drink or clean your teeth for 15 minutes before or after taking a remedy.

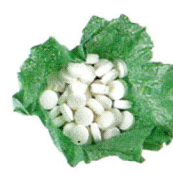

Homeopathic *Arnica* is an effective painkiller.

Herbal Remedies

To reduce uric acid, drink an infusion of gravelroot or celery seed 3 times daily. Steep 2 teaspoons of the herb in a cup of boiling water for 10 minutes.

Warning! If you are taking the medicine colchicine, do not try herbal remedies.

Acupressure

- Using your thumb, apply steady pressure just below the ball of the foot on the inside edge. Repeat on the other foot.
- Use your index fingers to apply pressure on each foot to the top of the webbing between the big and second toe.

Acupressure point below ball of foot

Chronic Pain

Symptoms

- Persistent muscle pain, along with swelling, stiffness and cramp
- Dull aching or sharp back pain, which is intermittent or continuous and localized or radiating
- Continuous joint pain and tenderness with restricted movement

Other related symptoms:
- Muscle weakness
- Numbness, pins and needles or tenderness
- Difficulty sleeping
- Lack of energy
- Depression

The broad medical term "chronic pain" covers any pain that lasts for more than 6 months, despite medical treatment. The pain can be mild or excruciating. Sometimes it can be difficult to diagnose the cause.

Causes
- Any of a number of conditions related to the ageing process, particularly ones that affect bones and joints, such as osteoarthritis, can cause chronic pain.
- Chronic pain can occur because of damage to the nerves from injuries or diseases that fail to heal properly.
- Chronic pain can be caused by poor posture or repeated movements.
- Having an injury such as a sprained ankle, or wearing high-heeled shoes can cause joint or muscle pain elsewhere in the body. Lifting objects in the wrong way or lifting heavy objects can strain the back and cause back pain. Being overweight can put strain on the back and the knees.
- Certain diseases cause chronic pain, including cancer, multiple sclerosis and peptic ulcers.
- Stress or other emotional problems can decrease the amount of natural painkillers the body makes, so increasing the level of pain felt. ▶

Alternative treatments

Aromatherapy
Mix together a few drops of the following essential oils with 2½ teaspoons of a carrier oil, such as sweet almond, apricot kernel or jojoba oil. Massage at the site of your pain, rubbing the oil well into the skin.
- To reduce inflammation and relax muscles, use lavender.
- To bring down swelling and speed up healing, try eucalyptus.

For a massage, mix essential oils with a carrier oil.

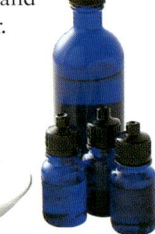

- To relieve the pain and stiffness of joint problems, try ginger.

Acupressure
Depending on where the pain is, a number of acupressure points can help reduce pain. Using the tip of your thumb or finger, apply pressure to the point for 1 minute.

Acupressure point above ankle for abdominal pain

WHAT YOUR DOCTOR WOULD DO

Your doctor will try to determine the cause of pain and treat you accordingly. For mild chronic pain, he may recommend over-the-counter painkillers, such as aspirin (though aspirin is unsafe for children). Stronger painkillers may be prescribed for more serious problems, and injections of a steroid drug may be recommended for some conditions.

Oral doses of an amino acid, D-phenylalanine, may be suggested; it may help your body release natural painkillers.

Your doctor may recommend going to a pain clinic where specialists will help you learn how to control the pain; for example, through meditation and biofeedback techniques. In severe cases, TENS, or transcutaneous electrical nerve stimulation may be suggested. This is a small device with probes attached to the site of the pain to block any pain signals. It is available for home use and you can apply the treatment yourself in the comfort of your own home.

Hydrotherapy (water therapy) can be effective in the treatment of pain. One type, for example, involves applying alternate hot and cold compresses to the affected area. Another involves swimming or other gentle exercise in a warm hydrotherapy pool.

SEE A DOCTOR IF

- You have pain for several weeks and it continues after taking over-the-counter painkillers
- Pain doesn't respond to medicine prescribed by your doctor
- The symptoms of your chronic pain suddenly change

- For abdominal pain, place your thumb on the inside of your leg, 4 fingers' width above the ankle. Repeat on the other leg. **Warning!** Do not use this point if you are pregnant.
- To ease pain in the upper body, place your thumb on the top of your forearm, 2 fingers' width above the wrist. Repeat on the other arm; repeat the cycle 3 times.

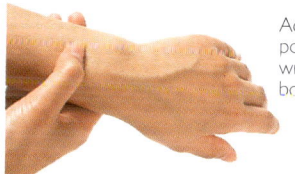

Acupressure point above wrist for upper body pain

HOMEOPATHY

- *Arnica* cream can reduce muscle and other pains not related to your joints.
- *Kali bichromicum* can reduce persistent pain and *Rhus toxicodendron* is good for back pain and pain related to joint problems including arthritis. Take 6c of any of these remedies 4 times a day for up to 2 weeks. Do not eat, drink or clean your teeth for 15 minutes before or after taking a remedy.

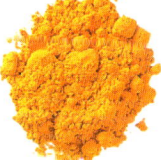

Potassium dichromate, the source of Kali bichromicum

Chronic Fatigue Syndrome

SYMPTOMS

- Fatigue, muscle pain and weakness
- Headaches
- Poor concentration
- Low fever and swollen lymph nodes
- Recurring sore throat
- Poor sleep

CALL A DOCTOR IF

- You are extremely fatigued with no identifiable reason

Warning!
Consult a specialist before taking herbal remedies – some of them can have adverse side effects.

Chronic fatigue syndrome (CFS) is the newly agreed name for myalgic encephalomyelits, or ME. It has many symptoms and can be difficult to diagnose; some doctors do not accept that it exists as a separate medical condition. It occurs most often in women under 45 although anyone can get it. The illness comes on suddenly and may last several years.

Causes
- No one knows what causes CFS, but research has shown that some sufferers have disturbances in their immune system. One unproven theory is that a virus attacks the body when the person is already fatigued or stressed. Other theories include antibiotics and body changes from exposure to pesticides or other harmful chemicals, or a food allergy.

What your doctor would do
There are no drugs specifically for the illness so your doctor will suggest ways of easing the symptoms, such as resting when necessary, taking exercise and making sure you have a healthy diet. Over-the-counter painkillers may help with aches and fevers in the short term. Some doctors prescribe antidepressants because, although there is no proof that CFS has a psychological basis, people with it may understandably become depressed.

Alternative treatments

Homeopathy
Treatments depend on the individual, so you may need to consult a registered practitioner. You can try *Kali phosphoricum*, which helps some people. Take 30c doses twice a day for 2 weeks. If your symptoms improve, repeat the dosage.

Aromatherapy
Try oil of lavender to reduce tiredness, weakness and pain. Put a few drops on a tissue and inhale. Alternatively, put 6 or 8 drops in a warm bath before you get in.

Acupressure
To reduce depression and fatigue and boost your immune system, try one of these pressure points.
- Using the tips of your middle fingers, gently apply pressure on the back of your neck at the hollows at the base of the skull, about 5 cm (2 inches) to each side of the spinal cord.
- Using the tip of your right middle finger, apply pressure about 5 cm (2 inches) from the base of your neck on your left shoulder; repeat on the other side. If you are pregnant, apply only light pressure.

Skin & Hair Problems

The skin is the largest organ of the human body. It protects the internal organs from outside invaders, such as germs and bacteria, and helps regulate body temperature through the action of sweat glands.

Although skin ailments are rarely life-threatening, some, for example blisters and corns, can cause discomfort, and others, such as acne or dandruff, can be embarrassing, particularly for adolescents. Conditions such as eczema and psoriasis are sometimes more serious and may need a long-term action plan for treatment. A wide choice of treatments can help ease irritation, and alternative therapies are sometimes particularly effective in dealing with skin problems.

Cuts & Bruises

Symptoms

Infection:
- Redness, swelling and pain
- A coloured discharge
- Fever
- Swollen lymph nodes
- Red streaks spreading from the injury toward the heart

Bruising:
- Discoloration of the skin: red, purple or yellowish green

See a doctor if

- Bleeding won't stop
- An infection doesn't soon heal
- There might be internal bleeding: signs include pain, weakness, faintness, pallor and perspiration

The skin protects us from infection, but can easily be cut or scraped. Bruising happens when there is bleeding under the skin.

Causes
- A cut, or incision, has a clean edge, usually from a knife or similar object. If the wound has jagged edges, it is called a laceration and the tissue is more damaged. If the skin is rubbed against a hard surface and is scraped away, the injury is called an abrasion.
- A bruise occurs when a part of the body suffers a sudden hard impact. It is normally minor, but very severe bruising can be life-threatening. Sometimes a bruise results from internal bleeding.

What your doctor would do
Most wounds can be handled at home. Wash your hands thoroughly, then clean the cut gently under warm running water, using a mild soap. Use an antiseptic wipe on the area, if there's a particular danger of infection, then dry the cut with a clean cloth or tissue. Gently press with a sterile dressing until the bleeding stops, then apply a clean plaster. Large or deep cuts may need stitching by a doctor.

To treat a bruise when the skin is unbroken, place an ice-pack, bag of frozen peas or a cold cloth on the area. Press lightly for up to 10 minutes to help reduce the pain and swelling.

Alternative Treatments

Homeopathy
- *Hypericum* 6x is recommended for painful cuts or severe bruising. Take 1 remedy hourly, for up to 4 hours. Do not eat, drink or clean your teeth for 15 minutes before or after taking a remedy.

St John's wort is used to make Hypericum.

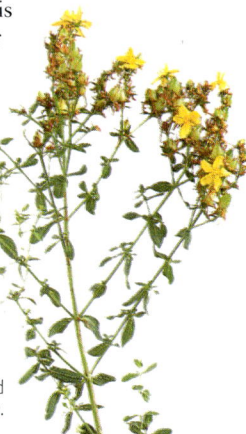

- *Arnica* is recommended for bruising. Gently rub the oil, cream or ointment into the affected area.

Herbal Remedies
- Calendula ointment acts as an antiseptic on minor cuts.
- Aloe gel is soothing and may help the healing process in minor wounds.

Aromatherapy
Tea tree oil is antiseptic. Add a few drops to water and wash the cut with it.

INSECT BITES & STINGS

SYMPTOMS
■ Itching and soreness
■ Red swollen bumps
ANAPHYLACTIC SHOCK:
■ Swelling around the face, lips or throat
■ Difficulty breathing
■ Severe itching, numbness or cramps
■ A rash
■ Dizziness, faintness or loss of consciousness

Warning!
If someone stung by a bee or wasp has the symptoms of anaphylactic shock (see above), call 999 right away! If the sting is in the mouth, get medical help.

Insect bites are tiny wounds in the skin caused by insects so they can suck blood. Insects inject venom into the skin to make this blood-sucking easier.

CAUSES
■ Insects that bite include mosquitoes, gnats, midges, horseflies, sandflies, fleas, lice and bedbugs. Ticks, spiders and mites, which are not insects but creatures known as arachnids, can also bite. In tropical areas, mosquito bites can cause malaria.
■ Stings are usually from bees, wasps and hornets. An allergic reaction to a bite or sting can cause life-threatening anaphylactic shock (see p. 30–31.)

WHAT YOUR DOCTOR WOULD DO
You can treat most bites and stings at home. Thoroughly wash the area with soap and water. Apply a soothing lotion such as calamine and avoid scratching the area. If it gets worse, see your doctor, who may prescribe an antihistamine.

If a bee's sting remains in the wound, gently scrape it out with a clean knife blade, needle or fingernail. Do not try to grasp it with fingers or tweezers. Then wash carefully with soap and water and apply a cold compress.

If you have an allergic reaction to bee or wasp stings, you'll need an injection of adrenaline.

ALTERNATIVE TREATMENTS

HERBAL REMEDIES
To relieve a sting, place a slice of onion or a fresh marigold flower, pulped, directly on the sting and bandage it in place.

Place a freshly sliced onion directly on a sting.

AROMATHERAPY
You can put 5 drops of the essential oil of eucalyptus in a cup of water and then rub the liquid on to the skin.

LYME DISEASE

A tick that lives on deer in the United States and Europe can cause Lyme disease, a sometimes serious infection. One noticeable symptom is a bull's eye rash that spreads a few centimetres away from the bite, but this is not always present. Other symptoms include headaches, fatigue, fever, chills, sore throat and aches – all flu-like symptoms. If caught early, doctors can treat it with antibiotics. If left untreated it can cause arthritis, heart trouble or other problems. Prevention includes wearing trousers tucked into socks and long-sleeved shirts in certain areas in the summer.

4

Urticaria ("nettle rash")

Symptoms

- Extremely itchy rash with white blotches on red patches of skin

See a doctor if

- Urticaria develops in your throat
- You have urticaria for a month or longer

Warning!
If someone who has been stung or bitten develops urticaria, experiences dizziness and has difficulty in breathing, call 999 right away! The person may be suffering from a serious condition known as anaphylactic shock.

A certain skin reaction, or rash, from an allergy is known as urticaria. This can occur when the immune system over-reacts to what it thinks is dangerous to the body. Urticaria usually disappears in a few hours but can last for a few days, depending on the cause.

Causes

- Some types of foods can cause urticaria: the most common culprits are milk, wheat, corn, citrus fruit, eggs, strawberries and shellfish.
- Certain drugs, such as antibiotics and aspirin, can produce urticaria.
- Insect bites or stings or contact with certain plants, such as the nettle, can cause urticaria.
- Urticaria can occur with exposure to heat, cold or sunlight.
- Emotional upsets and stress may also cause urticaria.

What your doctor would do

Urticaria usually disappears on its own, but in the short term you can apply a soothing lotion such as calamine. If it doesn't go away after a couple of days or you get it often, see your doctor, who may prescribe an antihistamine drug. Otherwise, try to work out what has caused the problem so you can avoid it in the future.

Alternative treatments

Homeopathy
Urtica 6c is recommended for itchy urticaria and *Apis* 30c for redness and swelling. Take a remedy each hour, up to 10 doses – do not eat, drink or clean your teeth for 15 minutes before or after.

Herbal Remedies
A fresh cabbage leaf has anti-inflammatory properties. Place it on the urticaria. Or remove the centre rib of the leaf, then pulp the leaf and place it on the urticaria; apply a bandage to hold it in place.

Apply a cabbage leaf to the affected area.

Acupressure
To fortify the immune system, apply firm pressure with your thumb on top of your forearm, 2 thumbs' width above the wrist, for 1 minute. Repeat on the other arm.

Acupressure point on the forearm

SHINGLES

In people who have had chickenpox, the viruses that caused it, *Herpes zoster* viruses, usually remain in the body but are dormant and do not cause any problems. In some people the viruses become active again at a later date, resulting in shingles.

Shingles typically occurs in elderly people but can also appear in young people. Symptoms last for weeks or months or, at worst, years. Shingles usually happens only once, but it has been known to recur in some people.

CAUSES
- Illness, injury or emotional stress weakens the immune system, which can allow the viruses to become active.

WHAT YOUR DOCTOR WOULD DO
There is no cure, but the doctor may prescribe medicine to help reduce the pain and inflammation and an antiviral drug to control the rash. Early treatment can prevent or reduce scarring from the blisters. If the area becomes infected, you may need to take antibiotics.

SYMPTOMS
- Pain, usually on one side of the body or face, followed by itching and a skin rash
- A strip or group of painful blisters
- A burning sensation at the site of the blisters
- Fever
- Generally feeling unwell

SEE A DOCTOR IF
- You suspect you may be about to have an outbreak of shingles
- The rash appears near an eye
- An infection appears
- You cannot bear the pain

ALTERNATIVE TREATMENTS

HOMEOPATHY
Take 12x of one of the following remedies every 4 hours for 3 days. Do not eat, drink or clean your teeth for 15 minutes before or after taking a remedy.
- *Rhus toxicodendron* to reduce irritation.
- *Antimonium tartaricum* to help the blisters heal.
- *Arsenicum album* for burning, itching skin.

Arsenopyrite is the source for *Arsenicum album*.

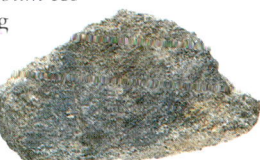

HERBAL REMEDIES
- A solution of lemon balm or calendula can be gently applied to the affected area to reduce inflammation. To make a solution, first make a tincture: half-fill a large jar with the herb and fill with an alcohol, vodka is ideal. Cover and leave in a cool dark place. Shake twice a day for 2 weeks; then decant into another jar. Mix together 1 part tincture and 1 part boiled and cooled water. The solution is now ready to be used.
- A commercial gel containing liquorice may help control shingles.
- Skin preparations containing St John's wort are often effective.

Blisters & Chilblains

SYMPTOMS
Blisters:
■ Bubble-like pockets in the skin filled with fluid; there may be one or many
■ Sometimes pain, inflammation or itching
Chilblains:
■ Itchy, purple-red swellings

SEE A DOCTOR IF
■ The blister results from a chemical burn
■ Blistering is caused by serious sunburn
■ If there is a discharge of pus

When the skin is irritated, bubble-like blisters can form. These may be the size of a pin prick or up to 1 cm (½ inch) in diameter or even more.

Chilblains are swellings that are usually found on the toes or fingers, although they may also develop on the nose and ears.

Causes
■ Brief intense rubbing of the skin can cause contact blisters. Wearing new shoes or ones that don't fit properly can cause blisters on the feet. Working with a hand tool can create a blister on the palm of the hand.
■ Burns and sunburn can cause blisters, as can certain chemicals.
■ Blisters may also be a symptom of an illness, such as shingles, or a reaction to a drug such as penicillin.
■ Chilblains are caused by the blood vessels narrowing too much in cold weather.

What your doctor would do
Most blisters heal on their own. If you have a troublesome contact blister and feel you have to pop it with a needle, make sure you sterilize the needle first, either by placing it in a flame or dipping it in an antiseptic solution.

Chilblains don't require treatment, although some people find applying unperfumed talcum powder to the area helps relieve the itching.

Alternative treatments

Homeopathy
■ *Calendula* ointment applied to a blister or chilblain can be soothing.
■ To relieve the pain of a blister caused by a burn, try *Cantharis* 12x, 3 or 4 times a day. Do not eat, drink or clean your teeth 15 minutes before or after taking a remedy.

Herbal Remedies
■ Aloe vera gel may be rubbed on to a blister from a burn.
■ For an antiseptic, mix 2 drops of chamomile oil in 250 ml (½ cup) of water. Apply to the blister; cover with a dressing.

Aromatherapy
Dab a little lavender oil on the blister.

Reflexology
If you have chilblains, you can improve your circulation by working on this reflexology point. Apply pressure to the heart point on the left foot, just to the side of the ball of the foot.

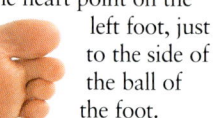

Reflexology point to the side of the ball of the foot

Sunburn

SYMPTOMS

- The skin turns red and feels hot and painful
- Dehydration
- Fever and chills
- Blisters may occur in severe cases, as well as nausea
- After a few days the skin will turn tan or brown coloured and may peel

SEE A DOCTOR IF

- You have blisters, fever and nausea

Warning!
Frequent sunburn, especially in childhood, can lead to skin cancer

The skin burns when it is overexposed to ultraviolet rays from the sun. Light-skinned people are most vulnerable, but dark-skinned people can burn, too. Sunburn usually appears 1 to 6 hours after overexposure to the sun.

Causes
- Exposure to direct sunlight puts you at risk of sunburn. The severity of the burn depends on how long you stay in the sun and where you are. Burning occurs more rapidly at higher altitudes and toward the equator and can sometimes take place after only 15 minutes in the sun.
- Sunlight reflected from sand, water or snow is just as strong as direct sunlight.
- Some medicines, such as certain prescribed ones to treat acne, make the skin extra-sensitive to sunlight.

What your doctor would do
For mild sunburn, apply a soothing lotion, such as calamine or a preparation containing aloe vera, and wait for the discomfort to die down. It's important to drink plenty and to avoid further sun exposure. For severe sunburn, the doctor may prescribe drugs to ease the pain. Hospitalization is necessary in extreme cases.

Alternative Treatments

Homeopathy
Cantharis 12x, 3 or 4 hours for 2 days, may relieve pain. Do not eat, drink or clean your teeth 15 minutes before or after taking it.

Coneflower is the source of echinacea.

Herbal Remedies
A cold compress soaked in a calendula infusion is soothing; steep 1 teaspoon of the dried herb in a cup of boiling water for 10 minutes. Or use an echinacea infusion on blistering skin to prevent infection.

AVOIDING SUNBURN

- Stay out of the sun if you can when it is at its strongest – between 10:00 a.m. and 3:00 p.m., especially in summer. If your shadow is shorter than your height, the sun is strong.
- When outside, wear loose clothes that cover your arms and legs and a wide-brimmed hat to protect your face.
- Use sunscreen or block on exposed skin. Make sure the sunscreen's sun protection factor (SPF) is at least 15. Remember to reapply it as necessary.
- Protect your eyes with sunglasses that give UV protection.

ACNE

SYMPTOMS

- Recurrent red swellings, or spots, on the skin, usually on the face, neck, back, shoulders and chest
- Dark pores, known as blackheads
- Infected, pus-filled spots
- Scarring may occur

CYST:
- Hard, inflamed swelling in the skin
- Occasionally infection
- Scarring may occur

Causes
- Acne is most common in the teenage years, particularly in boys, and is caused by an over-sensitivity to normal amounts of the hormone testosterone, present in males and females.
- People with oily skin are more likely to have acne.
- About one in five adults has acne. Women are more likely to have spots continuing into their 30s; these are usually more likely before a period.
- A woman may have a flare-up just before she reaches her menopause.
- Heredity may play a part.
- The contraceptive Pill can trigger acne, though one particular type reduces it.
- Other medicines, such as cortiocsteroids, can cause acne.
- A poor diet can aggravate acne; but only a very few people find that any particular foods make their acne worse.
- Stress can make acne worse.
- A type of acne can occur in newborns and infants, particularly in boys. It appears on the face and clears up within weeks, leaving no lasting marks.
- A cyst develops when a spot becomes infected and the infection goes deep into the skin. ▶

ALTERNATIVE TREATMENTS

HOMEOPATHY
Take either of these remedies in 6c doses, 3 times a day for up to 2 weeks. Do not eat, drink or clean your teeth for 15 minutes before or after taking a remedy.
- *Hepar sulphuris* is recommended to treat infected spots or cysts.
- Women can try *Pulsatilla* for spots associated with a hormonal imbalance.

Sulphur, the source of *Hepar sulphuris*, for treating spots

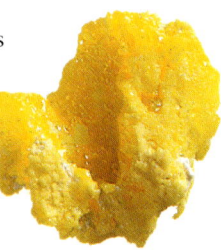

HERBAL REMEDIES
- A facial steam bath with fresh chamomile flowers or sage leaves can help open up pores. Making sure that

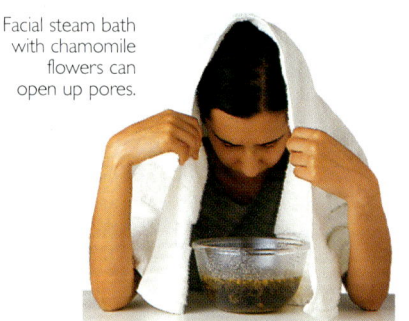

Facial steam bath with chamomile flowers can open up pores.

What your doctor would do

Many different treatments may help, including washes, creams and lotions which can unblock the pores and promote healing. You can buy over-the-counter treatments for spots or minor acne. Your doctor may prescribe drugs such as antibiotics, a certain sort of contraceptive Pill (for girls only) or vitamin A derivatives called retinoids in more severe cases.

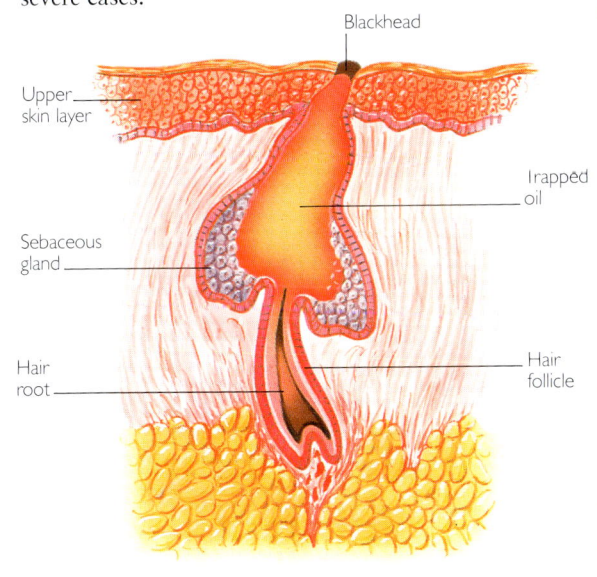

> **SEE A DOCTOR IF**
>
> - After using over-the-counter medicines for 2–3 months, the spots or blackheads don't clear up
> - Infection develops in spots or cysts

Blackhead
Upper skin layer
Trapped oil
Sebaceous gland
Hair follicle
Hair root

A spot develops when a small hair follicle becomes blocked by an oily secretion from a sebaceous gland in the skin. Just about everyone has spots at some time. There may be just a few scattered spots or many more spots over a large area.

the water isn't scalding, bend your head over a bowl of hot water with a handful of the herb of your choice, for no more than 15 minutes. Hold a towel over your head to trap the steam.
- Try a skin wash to reduce infection and inflammation. Using one of the following strained preparations, dab it gently on the affected area with cotton wool: a teaspoon of tincture of calendula (from a health store) mixed with a cup of water; a chamomile tea bag steeped in a cup of covered water for 10 minutes; a handful of fresh or dried yarrow, elder or lavender steeped in water for 10 minutes.

Acupressure

To ease inflammation, bend your left elbow and press your thumb on the outer edge of the elbow crease for 1 minute; repeat on the other side.

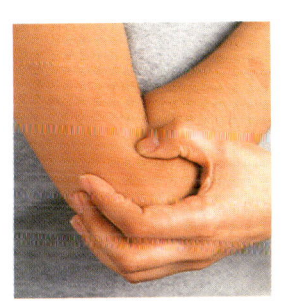

Acupressure point near the elbow, on the outer edge of the crease

DERMATITIS & ECZEMA

SYMPTOMS

DERMATITIS:
- Red, itchy skin
- Scales or, in acute attacks, oozing blisters

CONTACT DERMATITIS:
- A red rash where the skin has come in contact with an irritant

SEBORRHOEIC DERMATITIS:
- Yellowish greasy scales on the scalp, behind the ears, around the nose and on the eyebrows

ECZEMA:
- Dry, itchy skin
- Blisters and, later, scaling
- Thick patches on the wrists, face and creases of the elbows and knees

Dermatitis is a broad term for skin inflammation and includes contact dermatitis, seborrhoeic dermatitis and eczema.

CAUSES

- Contact dermatitis has many possible causes. Among them are some plants, such as poison ivy, poison oak, and certain garden plants; some fruits and vegetables, including oranges; household chemicals such as detergents, soaps and nail polish remover; and cosmetics and skin-care products.
- Wearing jewellery containing nickel, rubber gloves and new clothes before they have been washed can also cause contact dermatitis.
- Seborrhoeic dermatitis can lead to dandruff or, in babies, cradle cap. The cause is unknown but stress can aggravate it.
- Eczema is often associated with an allergy. The chief culprits are: cows' milk, eggs, wheat, nuts, dust mites, pollen, wool, detergents, and nickel in jewellery, cutlery and zips. Stress can also be a trigger. Eczema often runs in families and other family members may suffer from asthma or allergic rhinitis (hay fever). ▶

ALTERNATIVE TREATMENTS

HERBAL REMEDIES

Do not use any of these herbs for more than a month without consulting a trained herbalist.

- Infusions of dandelion or burdock can help eczema. Brew a tablespoon of the grated dried root in a cup of boiling water for 10 minutes and strain before drinking. Drink 3 cups a day.
- Evening primrose oil and chamomile or calendula ointment are good for reducing itchiness.

Warning! Do not use evening primrose oil if you are pregnant, have high cholesterol or have liver disease.

The root of the dandelion can relieve eczema.

ACUPRESSURE

Exert pressure for 1 minute on a point 4 fingers' width below the knee to relieve stress and strengthen the immune system.

Acupressure point below the knee

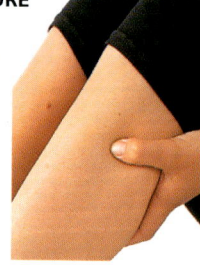

What your doctor would do

Treatments are aimed at soothing the skin. For mild cases, a bath followed by an application of an over-the-counter cream containing hydrocortisone is the first step. Your doctor may prescribe antihistamines, which combat allergic reactions, or antibiotics for an infection.

If contact dermatitis is suspected, or if it is thought that eczema is caused by an allergy, it is important to find the "trigger" – whatever it is that you are allergic to. Your doctor can do this by applying various irritants to your skin to see whether there is any reaction. One way to avoid some hand eczema is to wear white cotton gloves under rubber gloves when doing housework. Antibiotics may be prescribed for severe cases of eczema.

Moisturizing the skin helps many types of eczema. Unperfumed bath oil might help keep the skin moist. In extreme situations, a wet body wrap might be necessary; the patient sleeps in wet pyjamas covered with dry ones and covers his hands and feet with wet socks and his face with wet gauze. If you do this, don't let yourself become chilled.

SEE A DOCTOR IF

- There are signs of a skin infection, such as oozing pus
- The condition doesn't respond to over-the-counter medicines
- The sufferer is a baby less than 18 months of age
- You have eczema and come into contact with someone who has a viral infection of the skin, such as cold sores or warts

Reflexology

To treat eczema, a reflexologist concentrates on points which treat either the skin condition itself or the body as a whole. The point just below the bottom of the big toe nail is suitable if the face is affected by dermatitis. The reflexology point for the adrenals, which can help reduce inflammation and allergy, is located just below the ball of the foot.

Adrenals point just below the ball of the foot

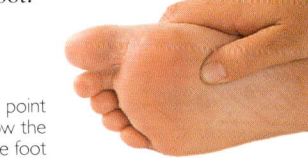

Face point at the bottom of big toe nail

Aromatherapy

Creams or nutrients containing essential oils of lavender or chamomile help reduce inflammation in some people with eczema.

Psoriasis

SYMPTOMS

- Red and inflamed itchy skin, usually with whitish silvery scales; in particular, on the scalp, elbows and knees, although it can occur anywhere on the body
- Discoloration, thickening and pitting of the fingernails and toenails; the nails may pull away from the underlying nail bed

SEE A DOCTOR IF

- The condition worsens while taking a prescribed medication or the problem persists

Psoriasis is a common skin complaint that occurs when skin cell production is abnormally high – about 10 times higher than average. This huge number of cells forms into white scaly patches, which can be uncomfortable and embarrassing. Psoriasis is rare in people with dark skin and usually appears between the ages of 10 and 40, although it can develop in babies and older people too.

CAUSES
- The cause is unknown, although psoriasis sometimes runs in families.
- Psoriasis may be triggered by illness, such as a streptococcal throat infection, stress, certain medicines or obesity.

WHAT YOUR DOCTOR WOULD DO
There is no known cure for psoriasis, but good treatment can keep most attacks under control. For mild psoriasis, your doctor may recommend taking a warm bath for 15 minutes to remove the scaly skin, then applying a preparation which helps the skin retain moisture. Certain drugs may help, including creams that promote the shedding of the scales and an ointment that prevents inflammation. In severe cases, the doctor may suggest steroid drugs or therapy in which drugs are taken and the skin is exposed to ultraviolet radiation.

ALTERNATIVE TREATMENTS

HERBAL REMEDIES
- Try an infusion of dandelion or burdock root or Oregon grape. Steep 1 tablespoon of the dried herb in a cup of boiling water for 10 minutes and strain. You can drink up to 3 cups daily.
- If the psoriasis is on the scalp, try a daily hair rinse containing dried rosemary and sage. Steep 25 g (1 ounce) of each herb in a 500 ml (1 pint) of boiling water. Let it stand overnight. Strain, and use it after shampooing.
- For itchiness, try evening primrose oil. Take 2 500mg capsules daily.

Warning! Do not use if you are pregnant or have high cholesterol or a liver disease.

AROMATHERAPY
- Mix 4 drops of the essential oil of juniper and 2 drops of cedarwood with a 1 tablespoon of almond or olive oil. Three times a week, cover your scalp with the mixture and cover with a shower cap overnight. Wash out the next morning.

Warning! Do not use juniper or cedarwood oils if pregnant.

Juniper is used to make an essential oil that can help psoriasis.

Corns & Calluses

SYMPTOMS

- An uncomfortable, sometimes painful, area of thick, dead skin on the feet or elsewhere

SEE A DOCTOR IF

- The corn or callus discharges pus or a clear fluid – it may be infected
- You suffer from diabetes, or any other condition causing poor circulation

Both calluses and corns are thickened areas of dead skin that form to protect underlying tissues. Calluses are common on the palm, fingers and the ball of the foot or the heel. Constant pressure and friction on the skin can result in a corn on a toe.

Causes

- Corns and calluses may be due to ill-fitting shoes.
- An awkward gait can also cause them.
- People with physically demanding manual jobs may develop calluses on their hands.
- Musicians who play a string instrument, such as the violin, viola, cello or guitar, sometimes have calluses on the tips of their fingers.

What a Doctor Would Do

A doctor may scrape off some of the skin to determine if you have a callus or a wart – a wart will bleed. A corn or callus will go away by itself once you avoid the friction or pressure responsible; but if it bothers you, it can be cut away by a doctor or chiropodist – a specialist in treating feet.

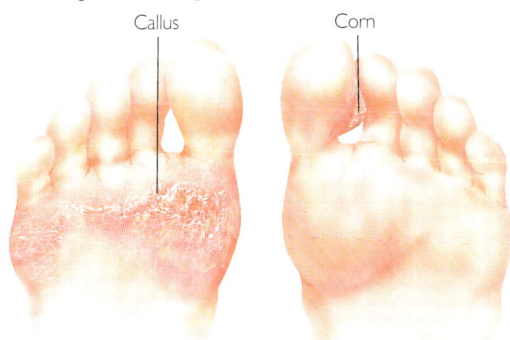

Callus   Corn

ALTERNATIVE TREATMENTS

HERBAL REMEDIES
- Apply a little calendula cream to the corn or callus to soften it.
- Crush a clove of garlic and hold it against the corn with a sticking plaster to protect and soften the affected area.

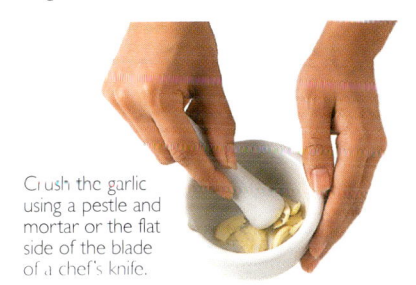

Crush the garlic using a pestle and mortar or the flat side of the blade of a chef's knife.

AVOIDING CORNS

- Wearing shoes that fit properly is the best way to avoid corns. Have your feet measured in the shoe shop the next time you buy shoes to make sure you are getting shoes of the correct length and width.
- Don't wear high heels all day, every day. Try to alternate your shoes so that you wear a different pair of shoes each day during any 3-day period.
- If corns are caused by the way you walk or stand, try wearing a special insole in your shoes.

Boils, Carbuncles & Warts

SYMPTOMS

BOIL:
- An inflamed reddish sore, sometimes with a yellow or white centre, that is painful and filled with pus

WART:
- A small, raised bump of hard skin on the hand, knee or face, or foot (called a verruca)

WART HYGIENE

- Don't share towels and face cloths if you have a wart
- Wear a plaster on a verucca if swimming
- Don't touch a wart or shave near it – you could spread it elsewhere on your body

A boil occurs when a hair follicle or oil gland becomes infected. A cluster of boils is called a carbuncle. Boils are most likely on the face, the back of the neck and the buttocks.

Warts are caused by a viral infection in the skin. A wart on the foot is called a verruca.

CAUSES
- A bacterial infection that enters the skin through a hair follicle.
- A contagious viral infection that causes warts. The virus can be spread by direct contact from the floor in moist environments, such as in showers and locker rooms or from shared bath mats or towels.

WHAT YOUR DOCTOR WOULD DO
Boils usually burst by themselves within a few days or weeks. If you have a carbuncle, see your doctor, or you may need a course of antibiotics to clear up the infection. Painful boils should be lanced only by a doctor to avoid the risk of further infection.

Warts usually go away within a few months but you can buy various over-the-counter treatments to help get rid of them. Because these contain harsh chemicals, they are not recommended for the face. If the wart doesn't go away, your doctor may burn it off using liquid nitrogen.

ALTERNATIVE TREATMENTS

HOMEOPATHY
Do not eat, drink or clean your teeth 15 minutes before or after taking a remedy.
- To prevent the infection in a boil from spreading, take *Belladonna* 12x up to 4 times a day.
- For a painful boil, take *Hepar sulphuris* 6x every 2 hours.

HERBAL REMEDIES
- Compresses made with comfrey, slippery elm or burdock infusions can help a boil come to a head. First make an infusion by steeping 1 or 2 teaspoons of any of these dried herbs in a cup of boiling water for 10 minutes. Soak a clean cloth in the infusion, wring it out and apply it to the boil.
- To fight off the virus, bathe a wart in tea tree oil or the juice from a dandelion stem.
- Apply a crushed clove of garlic or slice of onion to a wart and plaster it in place.

Chop a garlic clove, then crush it before use.

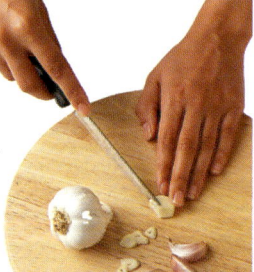

Athlete's Foot & Ringworm

SYMPTOMS

ATHLETE'S FOOT:
- An itchy red rash that may crack and peel, usually between the toes but sometimes on the sole of the foot
- Unpleasant foot odour
- Toe nails that are brittle and flaky

RINGWORM:
- A small red patch that grows into an itchy, ring-shaped rash

SEE A DOCTOR IF

- Athlete's foot does not respond to over-the-counter medicines after a month, or if the skin becomes swollen or weepy

Athlete's foot is a fungal infection of the feet that thrives in warm, moist environments and feeds on a protein in skin, nails and hair.

Ringworm is a fungal infection. It is not caused by a worm at all – the name is descriptive of the appearance of some rashes. It can be found in the groin and on the feet, scalp, nails and torso and is most common in children.

Causes
- As the name suggests, athlete's foot is common among athletes, who wear closed training shoes that provide the ideal conditions for the fungus to grow. It can also be picked up from skin particles shed in shoes and towels and on shower floors and around swimming pools.
- Ringworm is a contagious disease that spreads from infected people and domestic animals.

What Your Doctor Would Do
Athlete's foot sometimes clears up of its own accord; alternatively antifungal powders and creams that you can buy over the counter usually work. The most important advice is to keep the feet clean and dry, air them as much as you can and wear clean socks. In severe cases, the doctor may prescribe antifungal drugs. Antifungal cream or drugs may also be prescribed for ringworm.

Alternative Treatments

HERBAL REMEDIES
Tea tree oil can help ringworm or athlete's foot: rub it on the affected area daily.

AROMATHERAPY
For athlete's foot, soak your feet in a bowl of warm water with a few drops of tagetes oil.

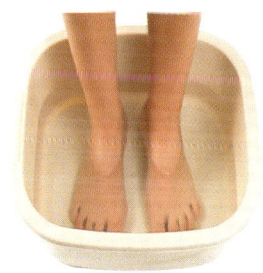

A foot bath with tagetes oil is helpful for athlete's foot.

SCABIES

Scabies is caused by an infestation with a tiny mite that enters the skin and lays eggs. It is usually found between the fingers, on the wrists and on the genitals. It causes grey scaly lines and is extremely itchy and infectious.

Your doctor will prescribe a lotion to kill the mites. Because they spread rapidly, everyone in your home should use it, even if they have no symptoms.

Wash all recently used clothes, linens and towels in hot water, and clean all your tables, chairs, floors and carpets. Put hard to clean items, such as stuffed toys, sealed in storage for a week.

Dandruff & Lice

SYMPTOMS

Dandruff:
- White flakes of skin on the scalp, often falling on to the shoulders

Lice:
- Itchy red spots in the affected area.

CALL A DOCTOR IF

- You have scalp irritation and thick scales despite regular use of anti-dandruff shampoos
- You have yellowish crusting and red patches along the neckline – this may be seborrhoeic dandruff, which requires treatment with presciption drugs

Dandruff is a condition in which dead skin flakes noticeably from the scalp; it is usually a little problem, although it can be embarrassing.

Lice are tiny insects that feed on the blood and leave eggs and small, itchy bites. There are three types, and they are all contagious: head lice live on the scalp; body lice live on the clothes and visit the body to feed; and pubic lice live in the pubic hair and are also known as "crabs".

CAUSES
- Dandruff can result from sebaceous glands producing too much oil, or from a fungal infection.
- Dermatitis (see pp. 66–67) or psoriasis (see p. 68) can cause dandruff.
- Lice spread when people are in close contact.

WHAT YOUR DOCTOR WOULD DO
Washing your hair with medicated shampoos usually clears up dandruff. In severe cases, your doctor may prescribe corticosteroid cream.

Head lice are best treated with twice weekly shampooing for two weeks. Each time, condition well to get rid of the tangles; before rinsing, comb carefully with a fine-toothed comb. This way you shouldn't need to use insecticidal lotion or shampoos. Body lice and pubic lice require insecticidal lotions. For pubic lice, treat sexual partners at the same time.

ALTERNATIVE TREATMENTS

HERBAL REMEDIES
- Both thyme and rosemary are effective in dealing with dandruff. Boil 2 heaped teaspoons of one of the herbs in a cup of water for 10 minutes, strain and cool. Massage the liquid into your scalp. Do not rinse it off.
- Massage tea tree oil into your scalp to help prevent infection.

AROMATHERAPY
The essential oils of rosemary and red thyme can be used to treat head lice. Mix 6 drops of each in 2 cups of warm water; use as a hair rinse after shampooing.

HEAD LICE HYGIENE

- Wash all clothes, towels and linen that may have been used by an infected person in hot soapy water and dry in a hot dryer. Soak combs, brushes and other hair items in hot soapy water for 10 minutes. Or place infected items in sealed plastic bags for 2 weeks. The eggs will hatch and die of starvation.
- Treat all the members of the family at the same time.
- It is a good idea to tell your child's teacher if the child has lice. The teacher can arrange for other parents to be informed, without identifying your child.

Women's Health

Women have certain special health issues, many of which are related to their reproductive system. These range from minor inconveniences, such as a craving for a certain food before menstruation, to major conditions such as the rapid loss of calcium from the bones that can occur after the menopause.

Children's Health

Babies and young children are susceptible to certain ailments that won't affect them when they are older, for example nappy rash and colic. Many complaints, although not serious, cause discomfort. But because the condition of young children can deteriorate quickly, all health problems should be professionally diagnosed if they last more than a very short time.

Bladder Infections

SYMPTOMS

- A burning sensation when urinating.
- A frequent need to urinate
- A feeling that the bladder still needs to be emptied after you have been to the toilet
- Strong odour from the urine

SEE A DOCTOR IF

- Cystitis does not clear up on its own accord within 24 hours
- You have a fever, vomiting, blood in the urine, or back or abdominal pain
- The burning sensation is accompanied by a discharge from the vagina or penis

An infection caused by bacteria that normally live in the intestines can lead to inflammation of the bladder, known as cystitis. Bladder infections are more common in women because their urine passage, or urethra, which conveys urine from the bladder, is shorter than that in men.

Causes

- Sexual intercourse can cause a bladder infection by pushing the bacteria up the urethra into the bladder. In some women, this happens every time they have sex.
- An infection can occur when a diaphragm is used for birth control. The bladder may not always empty completely when the device is in place, and the stagnant urine encourages bacteria to multiply.
- Pregnant women may get bladder infections because of the pressure of the fetus on the bladder.

What your doctor would do

If a bladder infection doesn't clear up in a day after trying a remedy below, see your doctor. He may prescribe antibiotics after giving you a urine test.

Preventive measures include drinking at least 2 litres (4 pints) of water a day, always urinating when you feel the urge, wiping yourself from front to back after using the toilet, passing water after sex and not using vaginal douches or deodorants.

Alternative treatments

Homeopathy

Do not eat, drink or clean your teeth for 15 minutes before or after taking a remedy.
- For strong burning, take *Cantharis* 30c every half hour, for up to 10 doses.
- *Staphysagria* 6c every half hour, for up to 10 doses, is good for cystitis brought on by sexual intercourse.

Herbal Remedies

- Cranberry juice fights the bacteria that can cause a bladder infection. Drink up to ½ litre (16 fluid ounces) a day to get rid of an infection.

- Or try an infusion of couch grass if you have an infection. Steep 2 teaspoons of the dried herb in a cup of boiling water for 10 minutes and strain.

Acupressure

Apply pressure just above your pubic bone for 1 minute, then gently massage around the area.

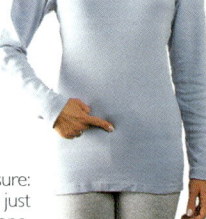

The acupressure point for cystitis is just above your pubic bone.

Thrush

SYMPTOMS

- Soreness and itching of the vagina and redness and swelling in the area
- A vaginal discharge that may resemble cottage cheese
- Pain during sexual intercourse

SEE A DOCTOR IF

- This is the first time that you have a yeast infection
- Your symptoms do not disappear after a week of treatment with appropriate over-the-counter preparations

Thrush is a yeast infection caused by a fungus called *Candida albicans*. It usually occurs in the vagina, but it is possible to get thrush in other moist areas of the body, such as in the mouth.

Causes

- It can be triggered by being generally fatigued, or sometimes by taking antibiotics.
- Diabetics are more likely to develop yeast infections because the high levels of sugar in their blood and urine encourage yeasts to grow.
- Although thrush can be passed on sexually, it is possible to get it without ever having had sex.
- Thrush is more common when pregnant or on the contraceptive Pill.

What your doctor would do

Effective treatments for thrush are available over the counter in the form of anti-fungal pessaries or creams. Thrush often has no symptoms in men even when there is an infection, so ask your sexual partner to apply the cream to his penis to avoid having the problem passed straight back to you.

In stubborn cases, your doctor may prescribe anti-fungal drugs.

Alternative treatments

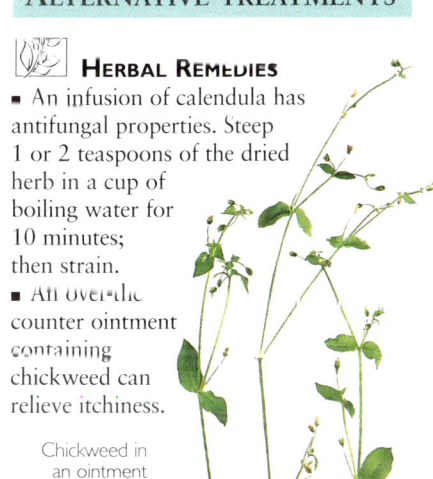

Herbal Remedies

- An infusion of calendula has antifungal properties. Steep 1 or 2 teaspoons of the dried herb in a cup of boiling water for 10 minutes; then strain.
- An over-the-counter ointment containing chickweed can relieve itchiness.

Chickweed in an ointment eases irritation.

SELF-HELP STEPS

- Eat a healthy diet
- Eating live natural yogurt may help replenish the bacteria that can guard against thrush. Putting yogurt directly in the vagina may be soothing.
- After you have used the toilet, always wipe from front to back.
- Avoid using perfumed products around the vagina, and don't put them in the bath. Don't use douches or vaginal deodorants.
- Wear white cotton underpants, which allow air to circulate. Avoid wearing clothes made of synthetic fibres, which increase moistness.

Premenstrual Syndrome (PMS)

Symptoms

- Irritability and anxiety
- Feeling tearful and depressed
- Abdominal bloating and tenderness
- Swollen, tender breasts
- Headaches
- Water retention
- Weight gain, up to 2.25 kg (5 pounds)
- Back and muscle aches
- Abdominal pain
- Fatigue or drowsiness
- Excess energy
- Nausea
- Diarrhoea or constipation
- Breaking out in spots or cold sores
- Craving for sugary or salty foods or for chocolate

The premenstrual syndrome, or PMS, is the name given to a range of symptoms that many women experience a few days to a week before a period. The symptoms vary: some women have only one minor symptom while others have a dozen or so. Sometimes the symptoms are so severe that a woman has to seek help from her doctor.

Causes

- No one knows precisely what causes PMS. Indeed, the medical profession is often at odds about suspected causes. There are many theories that may account for some of the symptoms.
- An imbalance in certain hormone levels can cause symptoms.
- A fluctuation in brain chemicals can trigger premenstrual syndrome.
- Dietary deficiencies, such as insufficient vitamin B_6, may be responsible for some symptoms, including fluid retention and bloating, tender breasts and fatigue. Stress can reduce the level of magnesium in the body, which is perhaps why some women crave food high in magnesium, such as chocolate. Low levels of essential fatty acids may affect mood.
- The premenstrual syndrome may have a genetic cause. Identical twins are more likely to suffer the same symptoms than are fraternal twins. ▶

Alternative treatments

Aromatherapy
- Place a drop of the essential oil of Roman chamomile or melissa on a handkerchief and inhale the scent.
- Add a few drops of the essential oils of geranium, clary sage and lavender to a bath for 2 weeks before your period.

Roman chamomile can help relieve PMS.

Homeopathy
Try *Pulsatilla* 30c for tearfulness and *Sepia* 30c for tender breasts, pain and mood swings. Take in the morning or evening a day before symptoms are due. Do not eat, drink or clean your teeth for 15 minutes before or after taking a remedy.

Acupressure
Press your thumb on the inside of your leg 4 fingers' width above the ankle for 1 minute; repeat on the other leg.
Warning! Do not do if you are pregnant.

Acupressure point above the ankle

WHAT YOUR DOCTOR WOULD DO

Your doctor may give you a general physical examination, as well as a pelvic examination, to rule out other possible problems. You may be asked to keep a diary of when your symptoms occur for a few months. This will help your doctor confirm a diagnosis and guide him in deciding on a suitable treatment plan.

There are few specific treatments for PMS. Some doctors may recommend taking certain hormones, perhaps in the form of injections or pessaries (tablets inserted into the vagina). Taking the contraceptive Pill or diuretic drugs to reduce water retention, can help reduce symptoms in some women. These methods, however, are not always helpful and may have undesirable side effects.

Evening primrose oil is rapidly gaining acceptance as a way of increasing low levels of essential fatty acids and easing PMS.

Lack of sleep can worsen some PMS symptoms, such as fatigue, irritability and mood swings, so it's important to get plenty of bed rest, at least 7–8 hours a night. If you have trouble falling asleep, sleep experts suggest establishing a regular sleep schedule, in which you go to bed and get up at the same time every day, including during the weekend.

SEE A DOCTOR IF

- Your symptoms are so severe that you cannot cope with your daily routine

HERBAL REMEDIES

- Dandelion leaves may help reduce bloating and swollen breasts. Skullcap can help alleviate nervousness and irritability. Make an infusion of either of these herbs by steeping a tablespoon of the dried herb in a cup of boiling water for 10 minutes, straining and sweetening with honey if desired.
- Chaste tree can help stabilize hormone levels. Make a tincture by half-filling a screw-top jar with the herb, then filling with an alcohol, such as vodka. Store in a cool, dark place for 2 weeks, shaking once a day. Take 10 drops each morning, starting 2 weeks before your period.

SELF HELP FOR PMS

- Cut down on sugar and salt, as well as caffeine and animal fats.
- Try a low-fat, high-fibre diet: eat plenty of raw fruit, vegetables, pulses, nuts and grains.
- Instead of having 3 main meals a day, eat small meals every 3 hours. One theory suggests that low blood sugar causes PMS symptoms.
- Exercise for at least half an hour 5 times a week.
- Take long warm baths to reduce stress and relax muscles.
- In the 2 weeks before your period, cut down on drinking alcohol.

Menstrual Cramps

SYMPTOMS

- Menstruation may be painful at the beginning of the period and for up to 1 or 2 days
- Blood clots in the discharge

SEE A DOCTOR IF

- You have a menstrual flow that is so heavy that tampons have to be changed within an hour
- You have sharp pain before your period starts or during sexual intercourse

Most women have painful periods at some time in their lives, most commonly between the ages of 17 and 25. This condition is known as dysmenorrhoea. It is often not as painful once a women has had a child.

Causes

- The pain is probably caused by the body producing too much of a particular prostaglandin, a hormone-like substance that makes the womb contract, in much the same way that it does during childbirth. Tightenings of the womb cause the muscle cramps.

What your doctor would do

Period pains are usually simply an unpleasant inconvenience that can be relieved with over-the-counter painkillers. But if they are very bad and stop you from going about your daily life for long, you should see your doctor, who may examine you to rule out a more serious problem. He may prescribe an ibuprofen-based drug or may recommend that you take the contraceptive Pill, which often helps.

Alternative treatments

Herbal Remedies
Cramp bark and chamomile flowers can help reduce period cramps. Steep 3 teaspoons of the dried herb in a cup of boiling water for about 15 minutes. Drink up to 3 times a day.

Aromatherapy
The essential oils of cajuput, sage, aniseed, cypress and marjoram are all recommended for painful periods. Mix a few drops of one of these oils with a tablespoon of a base oil, such as almond or soya bean. Starting 10 days before your period is due, gently massage the mixture over your abdomen and lower back each day.

Acupressure
Using your index fingers, press into the spaces between the big and second toes, angling the fingers slightly toward the second toe, and rub firmly before applying pressure for 1 minute.

Acupressure point between the big and second toe

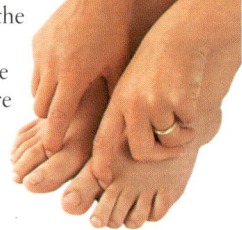

Heavy Periods

SYMPTOMS

- A flow that saturates a sanitary towel or tampon within an hour
- A period that lasts more than 8 days
- Large blood clots

SEE A DOCTOR IF

- Flow is so heavy that a tampon or sanitary towel is frequently saturated in an hour
- Your period is accompanied by sharp pain

Most women lose about 60 ml (2 fluid ounces) of blood during menstruation, but with heavy periods, known as menorrhagia, around 90 ml (3 ounces) or more is lost.

CAUSES

- An imbalance of certain hormones may be to blame as this may cause the lining of the womb to build up excessively.
- A disorder of the uterus, such as a fibroid, endometriosis or a pelvic infection, may cause heavy periods. Using an IUD as a form of birth control may also cause heavy periods.

WHAT A DOCTOR WOULD DO

It's important to see the doctor to find the cause of the problem. You may be prescribed hormones and painkillers as a first step. Iron pills may also be recommended if you have iron-deficiency anaemia.

If you still experience problems, your doctor may suggest a simple operation known as a "D and C" (dilation and curettage), whereby the lining of the uterus is gently cleared out under general anaesthetic. In highly severe cases, a hysterectomy, where the uterus is removed, may be an option – but a second opinion should be sought because this is a drastic and usually unnecessary measure.

ALTERNATIVE TREATMENTS

HERBAL REMEDIES

- Yarrow tea can control bleeding. Steep a teaspoon of the dried herb in a cup of boiling water for 10 minutes and strain. **Warning!** Do not take if you are pregnant.
- Shepherd's purse is used to regulate menstrual bleeding. You can make a tea by steeping a teaspoon of the dried herb in a cup of boiling water for 10 minutes, then straining it.

AROMATHERAPY

To provide relief from heavy periods, gently massage your abdomen in a clockwise motion with a few drops of the essential oils of cypress, geranium and juniper mixed with a tablespoon of a base oil, such as almond or soya bean.

Yarrow used in a tea can reduce menstrual bleeding.

Cypress, geranium and juniper essential oils are beneficial for heavy periods.

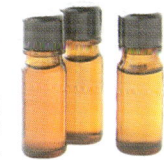

PREGNANCY DISCOMFORTS

SYMPTOMS

MORNING SICKNESS:
- Feeling nauseous or vomiting, usually only until the 12th week of pregnancy. Bouts occur in the morning and at other times of day

BACKACHE:
- Pain in the lower back that starts during the second trimester

HEARTBURN:
- Toward the end of pregnancy, an uncomfortable burning sensation in the upper abdomen, which is often worse at night

SORE BREASTS:
- The breasts feel tender and enlarged, almost from the start of pregnancy

Most pregnancies produce healthy babies at the end of nine months without any medical complications. During pregnancy, however, it is common for the expectant mother to experience a number of discomforts caused by the changes in her body. The most common complaints are morning sickness, back pain, heartburn and sore breasts.

Causes
- One theory is that morning sickness is caused by a change in hormone levels that occurs during pregnancy; it may trigger activity in the part of the brain that regulates vomiting.
- The increased weight of a growing fetus puts strain on the back.
- Heartburn is caused by acid reflex from pressure on the stomach as the uterus expands.
- Certain hormones prepare the breasts for breastfeeding by stimulating the development of the milk ducts and glands; these changes can cause a certain amount of soreness and irritation. ▶

ALTERNATIVE TREATMENTS

HOMEOPATHY
Do not eat, drink or clean your teeth for 15 minutes before or after taking a remedy.
- For morning sickness, try *Pulsatilla* 6c or *Nux vomica* 6c. Take either one every 2 hours for up to 3 days.
- *Conium* 6c and *Bryonia* 6c may help sore breasts. Take every 4 hours, up to 5 days.

HERBAL REMEDIES
To make an infusion, steep 1 or 2 teaspoons of one of the following herbs in a cup of boiling water for 10 minutes and strain if necessary.

- An infusion made from dried peppermint leaves may relieve morning sickness.
- An infusion of freshly grated ginger can also be effective.
- A chamomile flower or ginger infusion can help reduce heartburn when drunk after meals.

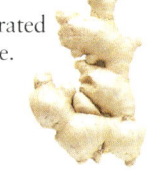

Grate the root of ginger to make an infusion.

AROMATHERAPY
- Add a few drops of the essential oils of lavender or geranium to warm bath water to help sore breasts.

What your doctor would do

These problems won't normally require a doctor's attention, but certain self-help measures will make you feel more comfortable.

- For morning sickness, eat small, frequent snacks instead of three large meals. Drink a lot of fluids too.
- To minimize backache, avoid putting on unnecessary weight: stick to a healthy diet and remember you don't have to "eat for two". Don't stand for long periods and avoid stretching up to reach higher places. Try to sit straight and make sure you have a firm mattress to sleep on. Bend your knees keeping your back straight when you have to lift something, and avoid lifting heavy items. Don't wear high heels except for once in a while.
- Eating little and often instead of three heavy meals can provide relief from heartburn. Try to avoid spicy or fatty foods. In bed, use extra pillows under your head so that your body is raised instead of flat, or raise the head of the bed a few centimetres (inches) by safely propping up the legs. If the heartburn is extremely uncomfortable, your doctor may prescribe antacids or other drugs.
- Sore breasts should be supported by the correct size bra throughout pregnancy. Rubbing on pure lanolin may help sore, dry nipples.

SEE A DOCTOR IF

- You have severe nausea or vomiting
- There is vaginal spotting or bleeding
- You have a severe headache, blurred vision, sudden weight gain or swollen fingers
- Backache with fever
- Blood in the urine
- Once the baby moves, the movements decrease or stop for more than a day

Warning!

Consult your doctor or a licensed practitioner before trying an alternative therapy. Some remedies have adverse effects on pregnant women.

- For morning sickness, add a few drops of the essential oils of chamomile or rose to a handkerchief and inhale the scent.

Acupressure

- For morning sickness, place your thumb 2 fingers' widths above the crease of your wrist on the inside of the arm. Massage in a circular motion for 1 minute. Repeat on the other wrist.

Acupressure point above the wrist

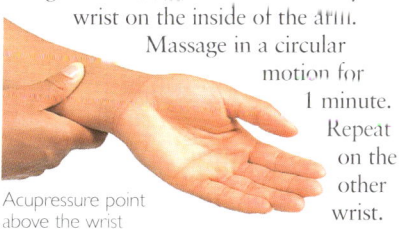

- Place your thumbs on your back, 2.5 cm (1 inch) on each side of the spine, just behind the navel, and press inward for 1 minute. Or rub the area with the back of your hands.

Acupressure points near the spine for back pain

Menopause

Symptoms

- Periods may become lighter and more infrequent before stopping completely
- Periods may be unpredictable for a while, with varying degrees of heaviness
- Menstruation may stop suddenly
- You may experience hot flushes – a sudden intense feeling of heat that spreads over the face and neck. They usually last only a few moments but may occur many times during the day
- At night time hot flushes accompanied by increased sweating may cause insomnia
- You may begin to experience vaginal dryness

The menopause is when a woman's periods stop altogether. This usually happens between the ages of 45 and 53, although it may occur sooner or later. When a woman reaches the menopause, she may have an increased risk of certain medical problems.

Causes

- Levels of the female hormone oestrogen decrease in the run-up to the menopause and can cause various symptoms which differ from person to person.
- The lower levels of oestrogen may have an effect on the health of a woman's bones; in some women they become so thin and brittle that a painful condition called osteoporosis develops. Women who are thin, have a light bone structure and have light-coloured hair are at a higher risk, as are women who smoke, are heavy drinkers or live sedentary lives. Women who have had anorexia nervosa in the past have a higher risk of osteoporosis too.
- The reduced levels of oestrogen may also contribute to an increased risk of heart disease. ▶

Alternative treatments

Aromatherapy

To improve your physical well-being, relax in a bath after adding 5 drops of the essential oil of sage and 2 drops each of the essential oils of cypress and geranium. Or, make a mixture of these oils for travelling, and when needed, sprinkle a few drops on a handkerchief and inhale.

An essential oil taken from the cypress plant is suggested for menopause.

Acupressure

To ease problems associated with hormone changes, press your middle finger on the point above the bridge of your nose halfway between your eyebrows. Apply gentle pressure for 2 minutes.

Homeopathy

Hot flushes can be reduced by using *Lachesis* or *Glonoine*. For either one, take 30x 4 times

Lachesis is recommended for hot flushes.

What your doctor would do

Hormone replacement therapy (HRT) may be recommended by your doctor. This can be effective in dealing with any symptoms of the menopause, and there's increasing evidence to suggest that it protects against osteoporosis and heart disease too. The therapy consists of raising your oestrogen towards its previous level. Because oestrogen alone can have serious side effects, such as uterine cancer, progestogen is often included. This hormone, however, can also have unpleasant side effects, such as headaches, bloating, breast swelling and irregular bleeding. Your doctor will discuss the benefits and problems with you before you decide on the best approach. The hormones may be taken orally or by skin patches or gels.

Your doctor will suggest you stop smoking as it lowers the oestrogen level. Increasing your calcium level may help prevent osteoporosis. Foods that are high in calcium include dairy products such as milk and cheese, sardines and salmon, broccoli, oranges and baked beans. To absorb the calcium, your body needs vitamin D. Being outdoors in the sun allows your skin to make vitamin D but always use sunscreen to protect your skin during exposure to sun. Half an hour's exercise five times a week helps prevent osteoporosis and is also good for your heart.

> **SEE A DOCTOR IF**
> - You experience vaginal bleeding after the menopause
> - Your symptoms cause you great discomfort
> - You have a high risk of osteoporosis

a day for up to 3 days. Do not eat, drink or brush your teeth for about 15 minutes before or after taking a remedy.

Herbal Remedies

A tea can be made using these herbs by steeping a teaspoon of the dried herb, or herbs, in a cup of hot water for 10 minutes and then straining it:
- You can combine chaste tree, wild yam and motherwort to make a tea for reducing the discomfort and frequency of hot flushes.
- To raise your oestrogen levels, drink black cohosh tea.
- A night-time drink to reduce sweating can be made by adding 3 drops of the essential oil of sage to hot water and honey.

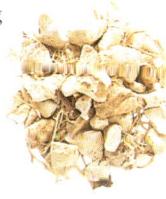

Wild yam is one of the herbs used to reduce hot flushes.

The black cohosh plant improves oestrogen levels.

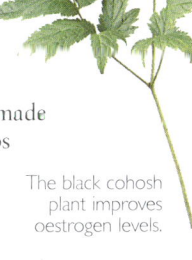

Nappy Rash & Cradle Cap

SYMPTOMS

NAPPY RASH:
- The skin is red and dry around the buttocks, genitals and thighs, and the baby may feel sore
- A strong smell of ammonia

CRADLE CAP:
- Yellowish or brownish greasy scales in patches or covering the whole head

SEE A DOCTOR IF

NAPPY RASH:
- The rash is severe or does not go away within a few days

A type of skin irritation in the area where a baby normally wears a nappy is known as nappy rash. Cradle cap is a type of dermatitis (see pp. 66–67) in babies that usually appears in the first three months, but it can affect toddlers too.

CAUSES
- Nappy rash is caused when a baby's skin is left in contact with a wet, soiled nappy, whether cloth or disposable, for too long. It can also occur if the baby is not dried properly after a bath, or if there is an allergic reaction to soaps or lotions. Sometimes nappy rash is caused by yeast or other infections (thrush), or psoriasis.
- Cradle cap results from the accumulation of dead skin cells.

WHAT YOUR DOCTOR WOULD DO
As soon as you notice any redness on the baby's bottom, wash it with warm water and dry it completely. Gently apply an antiseptic cream, followed by a barrier cream, and avoid using plastic pants while the baby has the rash. For a severe case, the doctor may suggest prescription creams.

To treat cradle cap, rub baby oil or olive oil into the baby's head, leave it on for 24 hours, then gently comb through before washing the hair. Otherwise, buy special over-the-counter shampoos.

ALTERNATIVE TREATMENTS

HERBAL REMEDIES
- Comfrey or calendula ointments can soothe nappy rash and cradle cap.
- To relieve cradle cap, add a few drops of tea tree oil to a mild shampoo.

AROMATHERAPY
Mix 2 drops each of the essential oils of sandalwood, peppermint and lavender oil in 4 tablespoons of a carrier oil, such as almond. Gently massage the mixture over the red area of a nappy rash.

Lavender essential oil can help relieve nappy rash.

PREVENTING NAPPY RASH
- Keep the baby's bottom as clean and dry as possible. Make sure it is washed properly and the nappies, either cloth or disposable, are changed regularly.
- Whenever possible, allow the baby to go without a nappy so that the skin is exposed to the air.
- To protect the skin from moisture, apply a barrier cream, such as one containing zinc and castor oil. Or use cornflour instead of baby powder or talcum powder (both of which can inflame broken skin) – as long as the baby doesn't have thrush, which thrives on cornflour.

COLIC

SYMPTOMS

- Crying spells that start when the baby is 2 or 3 weeks old, last up to 3 or more hours at a time and occur 3 or more days a week
- The baby draws up his legs while crying
- The abdomen looks distended and the baby may pass wind

SEE A DOCTOR IF

- You suspect your baby is colicky
- A colicky baby has fever, nausea, diarrhoea or constipation
- The cries sound as if they are caused by pain
- The baby is more than 4 months old and still colicky

Prolonged bouts of crying and irritability in a baby are known as colic. This occurs in about one out of five babies. Although it may cause frayed nerves in parents, colic has no lasting effects on the baby and usually disappears three months after it starts.

CAUSES
- Sometimes colic is due to a harmless but unexplained spasm of the baby's intestine.

WHAT YOUR DOCTOR WOULD DO
If the baby is crying more than usual your doctor can help you rule out any serious problem.

You should check for reasons why the baby might be crying. For example, the air might be smoke-filled and irritating. Look for an open nappy pin or a nappy rash that might be making the baby uncomfortable, offer the baby the breast (or bottle) to make sure she isn't hungry or thirsty, and to see if she simply wants the comfort of sucking or being close to you. Look for signs of illness.

Otherwise, try to soothe and distract the baby. Rhythmic activities such as rocking or a drive in the car can help, as can playing the static sound known as "white noise" from a radio that is set between stations. Wrapping the baby in a blanket or carrying her in a sling may provide a sense of comfort and security.

ALTERNATIVE TREATMENTS

AROMATHERAPY
To help relieve any discomfort associated with colic, gently massage the baby's stomach in a clockwise direction with 2 drops of the essential oil of fennel mixed into ½ teaspoon of a carrier oil such as almond or wheatgerm.

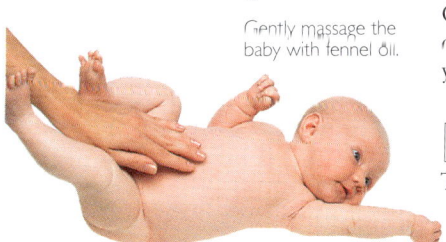

Gently massage the baby with fennel oil.

HERBAL REMEDIES
Chamomile or fennel tea may reduce wind in the baby's stomach. Steep a teaspoon of the herb in a cup of boiling water for 10 minutes and strain. Give the baby a teaspoon of the warm tea each hour but contact your doctor if the problem continues.

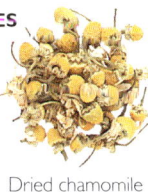

Dried chamomile can reduce wind.

ACUPRESSURE
To soothe crying, gently press the webbed area between the baby's thumb and index finger of each hand for 1 minute.

Mumps & Chickenpox

Symptoms

Mumps:
- Swelling of the salivary glands by the jaw joints, as well as fever, headache and difficulty in swallowing

Chickenpox:
- Itchy red rash all over the body and fever

See a Doctor If

- A person with mumps has a severe headache and stiff neck

Warning!
Never give a child under 12 years of age aspirin – it can cause a serious illness called Reye's syndrome.

Mumps is an infection that mainly affects children. Having it once gives you life-time protection. In adult males, it can cause the testicles to become swollen; if this occurs, a doctor should be consulted.

Causes
- Mumps is an illness caused by viruses spread by coughs and sneezing.
- The same kind of *Herpes* virus that causes shingles also causes chickenpox, a very contagious disease. It spreads by sneezes or coughs or contact with clothes.

What Your Doctor Would Do
There isn't a cure for mumps, but your doctor may suggest painkillers and drinking lots of fluids.

For chickenpox, your doctor may recommend taking painkillers and applying calamine lotion to the rash. Do not send an infected child to school.

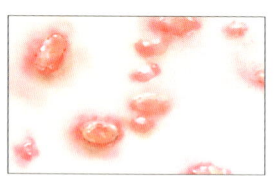

A chickenpox rash starts as spots on the chest and back. These turn to blisters and the rash spreads to the face, arms and legs. It disappears in 2 weeks.

Alternative Treatments

Herbal Remedies
- An infusion of calendula may held reduce the swelling of mumps. Steep a teaspoon of the dried herb in a cup of boiling water for 10 minutes and strain.
- An elderflower wash or a rosemary and calendula wash can soothe a chickenpox rash. Add 30 g (1 ounce) of elderflowers or 30 g (1 ounce) of each of the other 2 herbs to 850 ml (1 quart) of boiling water; simmer for 5 minutes. Allow the mixture to cool and strain it. Soak a cloth in the liquid and apply it to the rash.

Marigold is used to make a calendula infusion.

An infusion of elderflowers soothes a chickenpox rash.

Acupressure
To relieve the painful swollen glands of mumps, apply gentle pressure with your middle fingers in the hollows behind the child's earlobes for 2 minutes.

Measles & Rubella

Symptoms

Measles:
- Fever, coughing, red eyes, runny nose and rash all over the body

Rubella:
- Swollen glands behind the ear and at the neck; loss of appetite; rash in half the cases; and joint pain in an older child

Warning!
Never give a child under 12 years of age aspirin – it can cause a serious illness called Reye's syndrome.

Causes
- Measles is another viral illness that is common in childhood, but it can affect people of any age and is spread by coughs and sneezes. Measles can cause potentially serious secondary infection and inflammation.
- Rubella (German measles) is also caused by a viral infection that is spread by coughs and sneezes.

What your doctor would do
Always see the doctor for measles. He may advise taking painkillers and drinking lots of fluids.

There is no treatment for rubella, but if you have never had rubella or a rubella vaccination, and you are pregnant and have been exposed to it, see your doctor right away.

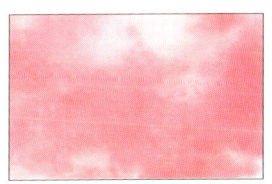

In measles, red spots appear near the hairline and spread across the face and to the torso. They then spread to the legs and arms and can merge to form irregular patches. The rash disappears after a week.

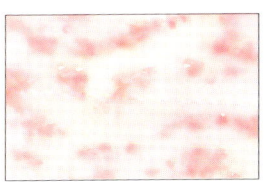

Rubella may cause a rash with tiny pink spots forming on the face and torso. After about 2 or 3 days, the rash on the face disappears, but a rash appears on the arms and legs and lasts for up to 5 days.

Alternative Treatments

Herbal Remedies
- For a measles rash, mix a teaspoon of distilled witch hazel with 250 ml (½ pint) of water and sponge on the rash.
- A cooled infusion of lavender can also be soothing. Steep a teaspoon of the herb in a cup of boiling water for 10 minutes; let cool and strain.

Diluted witch hazel soothes a rash.

At Home Care

Measles:
- Keep an infected child isolated while he or she is contagious: 8–12 days.
- If the child's eyes are sensitive to light, keep the lights dim and restrict television viewing and reading.
- To alleviate itching, apply a calamine lotion or a paste made with bicarbonate of soda and water.

Rubella:
- Keep the child home until a week after the rash disappears.
- Sponge with cool water to reduce a fever and soothe the rash.

Teething Problems

SYMPTOMS

- Irritability and increased crying at night
- Chewing on fingers
- Drooling
- When a tooth is about to break through, inflamed swollen gum
- Difficulty in getting the baby to take milk, either from your breast or a bottle

CALL A DOCTOR IF

- Teeth do not appear by the time the child is 12 months old

When babies reach about six months old, teeth that have been developing beneath the gums since before birth begin to break through. In all, 20 teeth should appear, generally by the time the child is 3 years of age. The speed at which the teeth emerge depends on hereditary factors.

Causes

- A tooth pushing through the gum can be irritating and may cause swelling where the tooth is about to emerge.
- The baby may refuse to take the bottle or breast because the mechanics of sucking bring blood to the swollen area, which increases the discomfort.

What your doctor would do

If the pain appears to be severe, your doctor may recommend special painkillers. Otherwise, you can only try to make the baby more comfortable. A cloth with an ice cube in it can be gently stroked over the gums. Some babies enjoy chewing on a cooled teething ring. You can also gently rub the gum with your finger.

ALTERNATIVE TREATMENTS

HOMEOPATHY

The following remedies are available in powder form to give to a baby. If the baby is still uncomfortable after a day, you should consult a practitioner.
- *Chamomilla* is recommended for teething problems.
- *Belladonna* is sometimes suggested for inflamed gums.
- *Pulsatilla* may also help reduce the pain associated with teething.

HERBAL REMEDIES

Syrup made from marshmallow root may help reduce soreness in the gums. Add 3 teaspoons of the syrup to the baby's food or drink each day.

AROMATHERAPY

To relax the baby, add 2 drops of the essential oils of chamomile or lavender to a vaporizer in the baby's room.

ACUPRESSURE

To help reduce the baby's pain, using your thumb and index finger, gently massage the web of skin between the baby's thumb and index finger. Repeat on the other hand.

Emotional Conditions

With the hectic pace of life today, many people struggle to balance their family life with demanding hours at work. While some stress is beneficial and necessary for good performance, prolonged periods of pressure can adversely affect our health, causing conditions such as insomnia and depression.

Other factors – relationship problems, for example, or a death in the family – may also act as triggers for emotional difficulties. And a lack of light during short winter days can lead to a form of depression, seasonal affective disorder, in some people.

While the prospect of developing one of these conditions may be worrying, they are not unusual, and the good news is that they are all treatable.

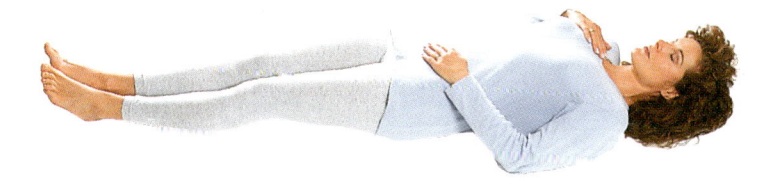

Stress

SYMPTOMS

- Headaches
- Fatigue
- Dry mouth
- Heart palpitation
- Insomnia
- Irritability
- Tearfulness
- Muscle aches
- Diarrhoea or constipation
- Skin rashes
- More susceptible to colds and flu
- Change in appetite, eating either more or less than normal
- More likely to worry about trivial matters
- Less interest in sex

Humans once had to deal with life or death situations on a daily basis when they had to protect themselves from predators. Our bodies coped with these situations using a "flight or fight" response, in which the heart beats faster, the pupils in the eyes expand and the muscles tense to help the body react quickly. Nowadays, the flight or fight response may become activated just by the strains of everyday living. A feeling of being overstressed occurs when we have difficulty handling these demands.

Causes

- An illness or death in the family can cause symptoms of stress.
- A break up of a marriage is stressful, not only in the adults, but also in any children involved.
- The birth of a child is often stressful.
- Moving can be very stressful.
- Pressure at work causes stress problems.
- Stress symptoms are often caused by financial problems.
- Positive experiences, such as getting married, buying a house or a job promotion can be stressful.
- Some individuals become overstressed simply by making everyday decisions, such as what to buy for dinner, what to wear to a special event or where to go on holiday. ▶

Alternative treatments

Herbal Remedies
Chamomile or passionflower tea can soothe stress. Steep a teaspoon of the dried herb in a cup of boiling water for 10 minutes, then strain.

Passionflower can be soothing when taken as a tea.

Aromatherapy
Put 5 or 6 drops of the essential oil of lavender into a hot bath and relax. Alternatively, add 1 or 2 drops of the oil to a hankerchief and inhale the scent.

Reflexology
Working on the reflexology point for the adrenal glands can help reduce stress, while the point for the solar plexus can help you relax. Apply pressure to these points for 1 minute each on both feet.

Reflexology point for the adrenal glands

Reflexology point for the solar plexus

WHAT YOUR DOCTOR WOULD DO

You may initially visit your doctor for one of the symptoms rather than the stress itself, but she may be able to diagnose the problem by recognizing the physical and psychological symptoms. Once the problem is identified, she may suggest ways of tackling the aspects of your lifestyle that are causing the problem. In severe cases, such as when coming to terms with the death of a loved one, an anti-anxiety drug may be recommended for short-term relief.

To help you cope with stress your doctor may suggest the following:

- Work out what is making you stressed. If you feel that you have too much to do, make a list of your tasks for the day, putting essential ones at the top. Learn to delegate some of the tasks and move less important ones to later in the week.
- Exercise makes the body release chemicals that act as natural anti-depressants. Take part in an activity you enjoy, perhaps with a friend.
- Don't rely on alcohol and cigarettes. They only make you feel worse in the long run. Try to eat a healthy diet and avoid turning to junk food.
- Take time out. Make sure you have at least an hour a day just for yourself. Go for a quiet walk, soak in the bath, or unplug the telephone and read.

SEE A DOCTOR IF

- You experience prolonged stress symptoms, as these can increase your susceptibility to certain serious disorders

VISUALIZATION

A progressive muscle relaxation technique can reduce stress. Each group of muscles is tensed and then relaxed from head to toe. It takes about 15 minutes and can be practised a few times a week while lying in a quiet room.

Take deep, slow breaths so that your stomach rises but not your chest. Tense each of the muscle groups for a count of 5, then relax them. Start with your eyebrows and forehead. For your jaw and face, open your mouth as wide as you can; then tense your neck and shoulder muscles. Lift your arms and tense them; then tense your rib and stomach muscles. One at a time, raise your legs and tense them and your feet. Lie still for a few minutes, imagining yourself in a special place, such as on a beach or in a wood.

You can listen to quiet music while practising the technique.

Insomnia

SYMPTOMS

- Unable to sleep through the night
- Waking up much earlier than normal
- Difficulty in falling asleep

Insomnia is the inability to sleep through the night and is an extremely common complaint. There are three main types:
- Transient insomnia: a temporary disruption of sleeping patterns that lasts for only a few nights.
- Short-term insomnia: a temporary difficulty in sleeping that lasts for a few weeks.
- Chronic insomnia: being deprived of sleep over a long period of time; this can have certain serious effects on a person's health.

Causes
- Travelling to a new place in a different time zone can cause transient insomnia. This type of insomnia can also be caused when your working hours change, particularly if you do shift work.
- Environmental factors can cause insomnia, including noise, lights or sunshine and a stuffy room.
- Poor sleeping habits may cause insomnia, for example, if you nap during the day or go to bed at a different hour each night.
- Insomnia is often caused by alcohol, caffeine and certain over-the-counter and prescription medicines.
- Stress and other psychological factors frequently cause insomnia.
- Certain disorders, such as heartburn, chronic pain and diabetes, sometimes cause insomnia. ▶

Alternative treatments

Homeopathy
Try one of these remedies in a 30c dose, 1 hour before sleeping. Do not eat, drink or clean your teeth 15 minutes before or after taking a remedy.
- *Nux vomica* is recommended for sleeplessness caused by anxiety.
- *Ignatia* can be helpful if you are suffering from grief.
- *Muriaticum acidum* is appropriate for relieving emotional problems.

Nux vomica can help improve sleep.

Herbal Remedies
- For a good night's sleep, steep 2 teaspoons of dried, chopped valerian root in a cup of boiling water and let stand for 8 hours. Strain, sweeten and drink before going to bed.
Warning! Valerian may impair your ability to drive or operate machinery.

The roots of valerian make a relaxing tea.

WHAT YOUR DOCTOR WOULD DO

Transient insomnia should stop once your body has had a chance to become used to any new routine; it normally does not require treatment.

For short-term and chronic insomnia, the doctor will treat the underlying problem causing your sleeplessness. She will examine you to look for a physical cause for the condition; for example, an overactive thyroid gland. If there isn't one, she'll ask you about any emotional upsets that may be stopping you from sleeping and may recommend a therapist. Sleeping tablets may be prescribed for the short term. Suggestions for helping you sleep may include:

- Go to bed only when you are tired. If you can't sleep, get up. Don't lie in bed tossing and turning.
- Make sure your bed is comfortable and that the room is warm or cool enough.
- Don't go to bed with a full or empty stomach.
- Avoid drinking caffeine in the evenings.
- Don't turn to alcohol; it can disturb your sleep and leave you feeling more tired in the long run.
- If you want a late night snack, eat a banana. This is a good source of an amino acid – tryptophan – that can relax and calm you.

> **SEE A DOCTOR IF**
>
> - You have trouble sleeping for more than a month
> - You are taking a prescribed medicine to help you sleep but it is no longer effective

---

- A tea made with chamomile or lime blossoms can help calm you. Add a teaspoon of the herb to a cup of boiling water and steep for 10 minutes before straining it. You should drink a cup before going to bed.

AROMATHERAPY

The essential oils of chamomile, neroli, lavender and rose all have properties to help you relax. Before going to bed, add several drops of one of the oils to a warm bath. Or sprinkle a few drops on a handkerchief and inhale the scent.

ACUPRESSURE

To help reduce anxiety and promote sleep, you can apply pressure with your index fingers to the points 2 fingers' width behind each ear and press for 1 minute.

Acupressure points behind the ears reduce anxiety.

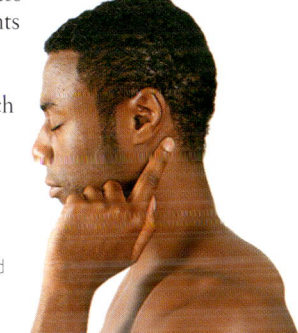

Depression

Symptoms

- Feelings of disliking or hating yourself
- Lack of interest and enjoyment in life
- Feeling guilty and blaming yourself for things that go wrong
- Extreme tiredness and lack of energy
- Insomnia or sleeping too much
- Reduced or increased appetite
- Lowered sex drive
- Thoughts of suicide
- Sluggish movements or speech

Everyone has days when they feel low or sad, due usually to some event or situation in their lives. In true depression, the depressed person not only feels low, but also has difficulty in coping with normal activities. A common illness that affects up to 50 percent of women and 25 percent of men at some time in their lives, depression has several categories:

- A depressive reaction is a type of minor, temporary depression that is a response to a specific life situation. It goes away in two weeks to six months.
- Dysthymia is also a type of minor, temporary depression but lasts for up to two years.
- Major depression is a serious condition that can lead to thoughts of suicide. It appears suddenly without a trigger and goes away just as suddenly, perhaps in six months to a year. It tends to be cyclical so it may return.

Causes

- A depressive reaction is usually caused by a major life event, such as death or a marriage breakdown; a reaction to a medication; hormonal changes, such as before menstruation or after childbirth; and illnesses such as a viral infection or chronic pain or fatigue.
- Dysthymia and major depression may be caused by an imbalance of certain brain chemicals called neurotransmitters. ▶

Alternative treatments

Acupressure
To help alleviate depression, use your index finger to press gently in the groove above the upper lip and below the nose for 1 minute.

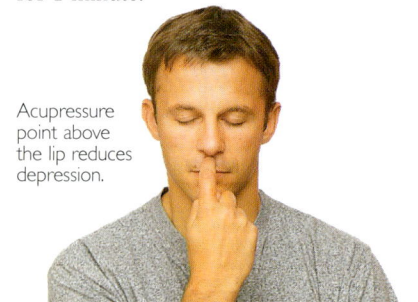

Acupressure point above the lip reduces depression.

Herbal Remedies
- Borage, St John's wort or vervain tea may help raise your spirits. Steep a teaspoon of the dried herb in a cup of boiling water for 10 minutes and strain.
- Rosemary tea can also help make you feel less depressed. Steep a teaspoon of dried, crushed rosemary leaves in a cup of boiling water for 10 minutes. Strain before drinking the tea.

Borage can help reduce depression.

What your doctor would do

Your doctor may prescribe antidepressant drugs. These have come a long way in recent years and some are often no longer addictive; indeed many people find drugs can be very helpful in getting them through a period of depression. She will also be able to put you in touch with a counsellor or therapist if you need to talk through your worries. She may also suggest you take some of the following measures to help you get through the episode:

- Try to involve your partner instead of trying to manage your depression on your own. Tell your partner how you are feeling. It may also help to talk to your friends.
- Get some brisk exercise for half an hour 3 times a week. Although it may be the last thing you feel like doing, physical activity releases endorphins – natural antidepressant chemicals – in the body.
- Don't turn to alcohol, cigarettes or junk food – they can make you feel worse.
- If you can, take a short break away.
- Remember what you used to do to give you pleasure and try to include these activities in your day to day life.

SEE A DOCTOR IF

- You or a member of your family has thoughts of suicide
- You or a member of your family has had symptoms for more than a few weeks

Reflexology

Several reflexology points help combat depression. Apply pressure to each one for 1 minute. Repeat on the other foot.
- Stimulate the 3 points for the head, which are located on the bottom of the big toe: at the base, the outside edge and the top of the toe.

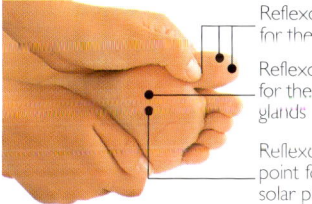

Reflexology points for the head

Reflexology point for the adrenal glands

Reflexology point for the solar plexus

- To aid relaxation, apply pressure to the solar plexus point, which is to the side of the ball of the foot.
- To reduce stress, press on the point for the adrenal glands at the ball of the foot, near the solar plexus reflex.

Aromatherapy

Essential oils of jasmine, bergamot, lavender, clary sage, rose and chamomile can be uplifting. Add a few drops of one of the oils to your bath, or put the oil into a bowl of hot water to scent a room. Alternatively, put a few drops on a handkerchief and inhale the scent.

Anxiety

SYMPTOMS

- Sweating
- Unreasonable sense of danger or worry
- Dry mouth
- Heart palpitation
- Chest pains
- Inability to concentrate
- Tense muscles
- Hyperventilation

SEE A DOCTOR IF

- You seem to over-react to a situation
- Anxiety gets in the way of your normal activities
- You feel anxious for several weeks
- You suddenly have severe symptoms

Most people have feelings of anxiety during times of danger or stress. But experiencing disproportionate anxiety or anxious feelings when there is no clear cause is distressing and debilitating. Anxiety comes in many forms: a panic attack is a sudden and extreme fear for no obvious reason; phobias are fears of common items, including spiders, schools, dentists, water, heights and enclosed spaces; and obsessive-compulsive disorders occur when anxiety and other emotions cause unnecessarily repeated actions, such as washing the hands repeatedly.

CAUSES

- Stress from an accident, illness, death in the family or financial problems often cause anxiety.
- An unhappy or frightening event that occurred during childhood, even though it is not consciously remembered, can lead to anxiety in adulthood.
- Anxiety may be an inherited trait.

WHAT YOUR DOCTOR WOULD DO

The doctor will examine you to rule out any physical causes, such as thyroid or heart problems. If nothing is found, she may advise you to see a therapist to get to the bottom of what is making you feel anxious. You may be prescribed anti-anxiety drugs, but these can be addictive so they are only recommended in the short term.

ALTERNATIVE TREATMENTS

AROMATHERAPY
Rub a few drops of the essential oils of jasmine, lavender or chamomile into the temples, or add them to a tissue and inhale.

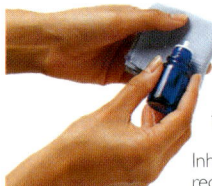

Inhale lavender oil to reduce anxiety

HERBAL REMEDIES
Steep a teaspoon of dried lemon balm, or dried chamomile or linden flowers in a cup of boiling water for 10 minutes and strain.

VISUALIZATION
Lying down, place one hand on your abdomen, the other on your chest. Breathe in so that you feel your abdomen rise substantially, while your chest hardly moves. Take 8 breaths a minute, then slow the rhythm. Once you have established a steady rhythm, imagine yourself in a quiet place, such as on a deserted beach or sunny hillside.

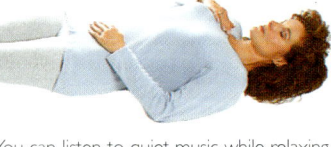

You can listen to quiet music while relaxing.

Panic Attacks

Symptoms

- Rapid and shallow breathing, or a feeling that you cannot breathe
- Heart palpitation
- Sweating and shaking
- Feeling dizzy or faint
- Numbness or tingling in the hands or feet
- Feeling nauseous
- Feelings of unreality and terror

See a doctor if

- You believe that you might have a panic disorder
- You think you might be having a heart attack – the symptoms can be similar

A panic attack is an unconsciously exaggerated response to fear, stress or excitement. Once such an attack has been experienced, people often become panicky at the thought of it happening again, so another panic attack can be triggered simply by the fear of having one.

Causes

- Panic attacks may be caused by a chemical imbalance in your system.
- Extreme stress – which may occur when a family member is ill or dies, or with a marriage breakdown – may trigger panic attacks.
- Some medical problems can cause attacks, as can certain medicines.

What your doctor would do

As with anxiety, there can be physical causes of panic attacks, so your doctor will rule those out first. If there is no physical cause, she will reassure you that the feelings, however dramatic and unpleasant, cannot harm you and will pass eventually. She may suggest that you see a therapist who specializes in panic disorders.

Alternative treatments

Herbal Remedies
Infusions made from skullcap, vervain or lemon balm can help soothe the symptoms of a panic attack. To make an infusion, steep 1 teaspoon of the dried herb in a cup of boiling water for 10 minutes and strain.

Aromatherapy
The essential oil of lavender is effective in relieving anxiety and stress. It is a good idea to carry a bottle with you; when necessary, place a few drops of the oil on a handkerchief or tissue and inhale the scent.

Acupressure
To relieve a panic attack, with your hand held palm upward, press your thumb firmly into your wrist on the same side as your little finger, about 1 finger's width into your arm. Massage the area in small circles for 3 minutes, then repeat on the other arm.

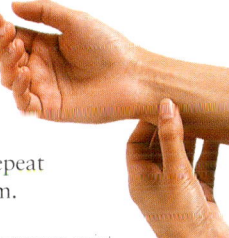

Acupressure point near the wrist can reduce anxious feelings.

Seasonal Affective Disorder

SYMPTOMS

- Depression; lack of enjoyment in life
- Lethargy and extreme tiredness
- Oversleeping and overeating
- Cravings for carbohydrates
- Anxiety and irritability
- Loss of sex drive

CALL A DOCTOR IF

- You or a member of your family experience any of these symptoms during the winter months

Also known as SAD, seasonal affective disorder is a form of depression that affects people during the dark winter months – it is also known as the "winter blues".

Causes

- What causes SAD is still a mystery but low levels of serotonin, a chemical in the brain, may be responsible. The levels are at their lowest in winter when there is the least amount of outdoor light.
- Stress and lack of exercise make the condition worse.

What your doctor would do

Many people seem to benefit from light therapy during the winter months. A special box that emits a light about 20 times brighter than normal indoor light is used by simply sitting in front of it for a number of hours each day. (Don't confuse this with a sunbed, which emits ultraviolet light and won't work, as well as being bad for the skin.) In some cases the doctor may prescribe antidepressants.

Alternative treatments

Aromatherapy
To relieve feelings of sadness, add 6 to 8 drops of the essential oils of clary sage, Roman chamomile or rose to a warm bath or place them in a bowl of hot water to scent a room. Or, carry a bottle with you; when needed, put a drop on a handkerchief and inhale the scent.

Homeopathy
If you are feeling weepy and sad, you can try *Pulsatilla* 6c. Take it 3 times a day, for up to 2 weeks. Do not eat, drink or brush your teeth for 15 minutes before or after taking a remedy.

Wintertime self-help

- Try to spend some time outside in the daylight each day.
- Go outside in the middle of the day for a 30-minute walk, even if it is a cloudy day.
- Try to work in front of a window. If necessary, trim any tree branches and shrubs near the window to allow as much light in as possible.
- Consider taking a holiday during winter in a place with longer days and brighter sun.

ALTERNATIVE HEALTH

Many treatments in conventional medicine are directly related to the principles of some alternative health therapies. For example, like herbal remedies, aspirin was originally derived from a plant, and homeopathy and vaccination may prove to work on roughly similar principles.

Today, alternative therapies are often used to complement conventional medicine. Some, such as herbal remedies and acupressure, have been around for thousands of years; others, for example reflexology, are relatively new, but their proponents are firm believers in the results.

If you fall ill, it is always best to see your doctor first, but you can use alternative therapies to alleviate symptoms alongside your doctor's recommendations – as long as you remember to inform your practitioner of your medical diagnosis and your doctor about any remedies you are taking.

Homeopathy

How it works

Homeopathy is a system of medicine developed in the 1790s by the German physician Samuel Hahnemann. He noticed that a herbal remedy for malaria (which was later found to contain quinine – the first medicine used to treat malaria) produced the same symptoms in a healthy person as malaria. He deduced that the symptoms were nature's way of fighting the disease – a theory expressed by the Greek physician Hippocrates 2,300 years earlier. So homeopathy is based on the idea of curing "like with like". In other words, elements that can cause the symptoms of a particular illness can, in the right doses, be used to cure it. Vaccines work on this principle: they are made from dead or live viruses and, when injected, provide immunity to the disease itself.

The effectiveness of homeopathy is still debated, but the few studies that there are show that it probably can help certain conditions, including hay fever, asthma and flu.

What to expect from a practitioner

Homeopaths focus on the whole patient, not just the illness. They consider a person's mental, physical and emotional traits along with the ailment.

A trained homeopath, who often has prior medical training, takes a patient's complete physical and psychological history in order to work out the most effective treatment. He then prescribes remedies in the form of little pills, called pillules, powders, creams or tinctures to be taken over a short period of time. If these don't have the desired effect, he may make another diagnosis.

Can I treat myself?

Although it is best to seek help from a professional homeopath for any chronic or serious disease or disorder, remedies for common short-term illnesses are available from many pharmacists and health food stores or, if necessary, from a specialist homeopathic pharmacy – ask your pharmacist for details. Homeopathic medicines are safe for people of all ages, but you should take them only for as long as needed. Inform your homeopath if you are taking conventional medicine as well.

THE MAKING OF A REMEDY

A remedy is made by soaking a substance – such as a plant, mineral or insect – in alcohol to extract the active ingredients. The solution is then diluted numerous times. It is believed that the more the solution is diluted, the more powerful it becomes.

A "c" after a number means that a remedy has been diluted 100 times multiplied by the number; an "x", 10 times multiplied by the number. So a 6c dose has been diluted 600 times and is therefore much more powerful than a 6x dose, which has been diluted only 60 times.

TAKING A REMEDY

A remedy should be touched only by the person taking it, and then as little as possible; don't take one that has been dropped. For best results, do not eat, drink or clean your teeth for 15 minutes before or after taking it. Some remedies are placed under the tongue and sucked; others can be chewed.

Homeopathy First Aid Kit

You can take the appropriate remedy every 2 hours for up to 6 doses. For information on doses and taking a remedy, see the boxes on the opposite page.

Source	Used for
Apis 30c from bees, pollen, honey and beeswax	Allergic reactions in the eyes, throat and mouth; sore throats; urticaria; cystitis; and insect stings. **Warning!** Do not use if pregnant.
Arnica 6c or 30c from *Arnica montana* (leopard's bane)	Burns; stings; bruising; black eyes; nose bleeds; cuts and abrasions; cramp; sprains and strained muscles; arthritis; shock after injury; eczema; and whooping cough.
Bryonia 30c from the root of *Bryonia alba* (common bryony, wild hops)	Headaches; colds and flu; nausea; heat exhaustion; painful breasts; and arthritis.
Cantharis 6c or 30c from a secretion made by the beetle called Spanish fly	Burns and scalds; blisters; burning or stinging sensations; and cystitis.
Euphrasia 6c from *Euphrasia officinalis* (eyebright)	Conjunctivitis; eyestrain or eye injuries; and constipation.
Hypericum 30c from *Hypericum* (St John's wort)	Cuts and abrasions; discomfort after dental treatment; head wounds; wounds with shooting pains; injuries that affect the nerves; depression; indigestion; nausea; and diarrhoea.
Nux vomica 6c from *Strychnos nux vomica* (poison nut tree)	Colds and flu; heavy periods; morning sickness; labour pains; frequent urination in pregnancy; cystitis, travel sickness; digestive problems; hangovers; insomnia.
Silicea 6c from the mineral silica, found in many rocks	Recurring colds and infections; spots; and migraine.
Tabacum 6c from *Nicotiana tabacum* (the tobacco plant)	Nausea and vomiting; travel sickness; faintness and dizziness; and anxiety.
Urtica 6c from *Urtica urens* (dwarf stinging nettle)	Burns and scalds; urticaria and other skin allergies; and cystitis.

Herbal Remedies

Making an Infusion

To make a herbal infusion, or tea, put 1 or 2 teaspoons of the dried herb into a cup. Fill the cup with boiling water and steep, or let stand, for 10 minutes. Strain the tea, then add honey or sugar to mask any bitter or unpleasant taste.

If using fresh herbs, use 2 to 4 teaspoons. To make larger quantities, use 15–30g (½ to 1 ounce) of dried herb (double the amount of fresh herb) for every 600ml (2 cups) of water. Teas lose their medicinal qualities when exposed to air for a few hours. Store in a tightly sealed jar in the refrigerator for up to 3 days and warm gently when needed.

Warning!
Pregnant and breast-feeding women should consult a qualified herbal medicine practitioner before taking any herbal remedy. There are some herbs which should **never** be taken in pregnancy.

How They Work

A variety of plant parts – flowers, fruit, leaves, roots, stems, bark and seeds – are used to prepare herbal medicines. These contain ingredients that can help heal, cure or relieve symptoms. Herbal medicine is one of the oldest forms of medicine. The slaves who built the pyramids in Egypt thousands of years ago took garlic every day to avoid catching infections. Today, about one quarter of conventional medicines include some type of active ingredient derived from plants. Herbal remedies often taken longer to work than conventional medicine, partly because they are used in less concentrated forms.

What to Expect from a Practitioner

Instead of treating a symptom directly, herbalists try to restore what they call the vital force – the body's own healing ability. A practitioner will ask about your lifestyle, diet and emotional state before choosing a remedy, and will also want to know about your medical history and any conventional medicines that you may be taking. The remedy will then be prescribed in the lowest dose that will work.

Herbal remedies can be found in health food stores or specialist shops. They are sold as tea bags; pills, capsules and powders; extracts and tinctures – types of concentrated liquids; and lotions, creams and ointments. Herbs are also available for making your own teas (or infusions), compresses, poultices, tinctures and ointments at home. Herbs are best absorbed on an empty stomach. If a herb makes you feel nauseous, take it with a meal. If headaches, diarrhoea or nausea consistently occur within 2 hours, tell your herbalist, who will change the remedy.

Can I Treat Myself?

The most effective treatments for serious or chronic conditions are best prescribed by a qualified herbal medicine practitioner. In general, herbal remedies should be discussed with a practitioner because some herbs can be toxic if taken in the wrong concentrations. You can buy some of your own remedies, however, for certain common minor illnesses but consult your doctor if the symptoms persist or worsen, or if new ones appear, or if you are taking any conventional medicine.

COMMON HERBAL REMEDIES

These herbs can easily be found in health food stores, and the remedies can safely be used at home.

HERB	USES
Burdock Arctium lappa	**As a compress**: use on cuts and abrasions. Soak a cloth in burdock tea before applying to the wound. **As a decoction**: take for fungal and bacterial infections; eczema and psoriasis; cystitis; and arthritis. Boil 1 teaspoon of the chopped root in 3 cups water for 30 minutes.
Calendula Calendula officinalis	**As an infusion** (see opposite): take 2 to 4 times daily for indigestion and period problems. Do not use if pregnant. **As a lotion or ointment**: rub on cuts and abrasions; measles and chickenpox rashes; and nappy rash and athlete's foot.
German chamomile Chamomilla recutita (also known as Matricaria recutita)	**As an infusion of the flowers** (see opposite): take 3 to 4 times daily for indigestion; menstrual cramps and colic; and just before bedtime for insomnia. **As a compress**: use for swelling, painful joints; inflamed skin and sunburn; cuts and abrasions; haemorrhoids; and sore eyes. Soak the cloth in a strained infusion at room temperature diluted with an equal part of water.
Comfrey Symphytum officinale	**As a poultice**: for cuts and abrasions; insect bites; bruises; and inflamed skin. Shake the powder over the affected area and cover with a clean cloth or plaster.
Eyebright Euphrasia officinalis	**As an infusion** (see opposite): drink 3 cups daily for stuffy noses; coughs from colds; sinusitis; and allergies. **As a compress**: apply to eyes irritated by hay fever or other allergies; colds; and conjunctivitis. Dip a clean cloth in a strained infusion at room temperature; apply for 15 minutes.
Hyssop Hyssopus officinalis	**As an infusion** (see opposite): drink 3 times a day for colds, coughs and bronchitis; indigestion and gas; and anxiety. **As a compress** (soak a clean cloth in 2 batches of the infusion): use for cold sores; burns; cuts; and other skin irritations.
Lavender Lavandula officinalis	**As an infusion** (see opposite): drink 3 times a day for insomnia or depression; headache; stress; indigestion; nausea; and flatulence.
Stinging nettle Urtica dioica	**As an infusion** (see opposite): drink 2 times a day for hay fever; eczema; thrush; premenstrual syndrome; heavy periods; diarrhoea; cystitis; haemorrhoids; arthritis; and gout.

AROMATHERAPY

MASSAGE

Add a few drops of essential oil to a teaspoon of a carrier oil, such as almond or soya, and massage it into the skin. For a back massage a teaspoon is enough. You can massage the parts of your body you can reach, rubbing the oil into your skin, but you'll need someone else to give you a full body massage.

OTHER WAYS TO USE THE OILS

- In the bath: add about 5 drops of the essential oil to a warm bath water, stir and settle down and relax.
- As a compress: add 4–5 drops to a bowl of water. Soak a clean cloth in it, picking up as much of the oil as you can; wring it out and apply to the affected area. Use hot water for muscle pain and arthritis, cold water for headaches, sprains and swellings.
- As an inhalation: put 3–4 drops in a bowl of hot water and bend your head over the bowl and cover it with a towel. Or put a few drops on a clean handkerchief and inhale the aroma.

How it works

The oil extracted from certain plants is believed to have the ability to relax people and relieve the symptoms of certain disorders. This practise of using essential oils has been a part of human history for thousands of years. In fact, ancient Chinese documents describe the importance that aromas play in promoting both physical health and spirituality.

The fragrance of the essential oils affects the part of the brain that controls memory, emotion and hormone levels. Some oils are also absorbed through the skin and carried throughout the body by the bloodstream and lymph. In particular, the oils can benefit muscular pains; digestive disorders; symptoms of menstruation and the menopause; stress-related problems; depression; and insomnia.

What to expect from a practitioner

The practitioner will usually begin the first visit by asking you a series of questions about yourself and your problem. This information helps her to find out about your general health and lifestyle, including your diet, exercise, posture and sleeping habits. A selection of essential oils will be chosen and blended together. The mixture will be given to you to take home. The practitioner may also give you a massage treatment during the visit.

Can I treat myself?

You can use the essential oils at home for certain common disorders and they can be used combined. You should always buy high-quality oils from a specialist supplier to make sure you get pure essential oils. Unless you are using tree tea oil, don't apply the oil directly to your skin – the oils are concentrated and can cause irritation. There are many ways to use the oils, including massage, in a bath, inhaling and as a compress (see left). Sometimes essential oils may be recommended as a gargle, but unless you are following instructions from a practitioner, this should not be practised because it can be dangerous.

Warning! If you are pregnant, always consult a practitioner first – there are a number of oils that pregnant women should avoid.

COMMON ESSENTIAL OILS

Below are some suggestions for using common essential oils. Although certain methods of using an oil for particular conditions are given below, others may also be appropriate. For ways of using the oils, see the boxes on the opposite page.

ESSENTIAL OILS	USES
Chamomile *Chamomilla recutita* and *Chamomilla nobile* (also known as *Matricaria recutita* and *Matricaria nobile*)	**As a massage:** for menstrual cramps and heavy periods; muscle pain and arthritic pain; insomnia, anxiety and stress; and indigestion and flatulence. **In a bath:** for stress, anxiety and insomnia. **With a few drops on cottonwool:** dab on acne, eczema, cuts and abrasions.
Eucalyptus *Eucalyptus globulus*	**In an inhalation:** for coughs, colds, flu, sinusitis and bronchitis. **As a massage:** good for muscle aches and fibrositis. **On a compress:** soothes insect bites and rashes from chickenpox or shingles. **With a few drops on cottonwool:** dab on cuts, abrasions, bruises and burns.
Lavender *Lavandula angustifolia*	**As a massage:** for muscle aches; colic; stomach ache, nausea, indigestion and flatulence; and stress, depression and insomnia. **In a bath:** for stress, depression and insomnia. **In an inhalation:** for catarrh, colds, flu and bronchitis. **On a compress:** for burns, bruises, acne, urticaria and insect bites.
Rosemary *Romarinus officinalis*	**As a massage:** for muscle aches and strains; menstrual cramps; and fluid retention. **In an inhalation:** for colds, coughs, catarrh and headaches. **On a compress:** for muscle aches; sprains; headaches; indigestion; and flatulence. **In a bath:** for menstrual cramps and fluid retention.
Tea tree *Melaleuca alternifolia*	**Applied directly to the skin:** for cuts, insect stings, cold sores, mouth ulcers and warts. **In an inhalation:** for colds, flu and sinusitis. **On a compress:** for blisters; rashes from chickenpox and shingles; and other rashes.

ACUPRESSURE

APPLYING PRESSURE

To apply pressure to a point, use the tip of your finger, not the nail. Place it on the point (it should make a slight depression) and press lightly. Increase the pressure until it is firm, yet comfortable. Hold the pressure until you feel your pulse; some people feel a sensation.

HOW IT WORKS

One of a number of treatments used in traditional Chinese medicine, acupressure is based on applying pressure to precise points on the body to strengthen, calm or unblock the flow of "chi", or vital energy. These points are located on meridians – pathways in the body, said to correspond with blood vessels or nerves. There are two sets of 12 meridians that run along each side of the body and have the same points. Two additional meridians run down the centre of the body. By applying pressure to a point, a particular symptom can be relieved; pressing several points in a certain order can improve the well-being of the body as a whole. Research has shown that acupressure relieves nausea and pain.

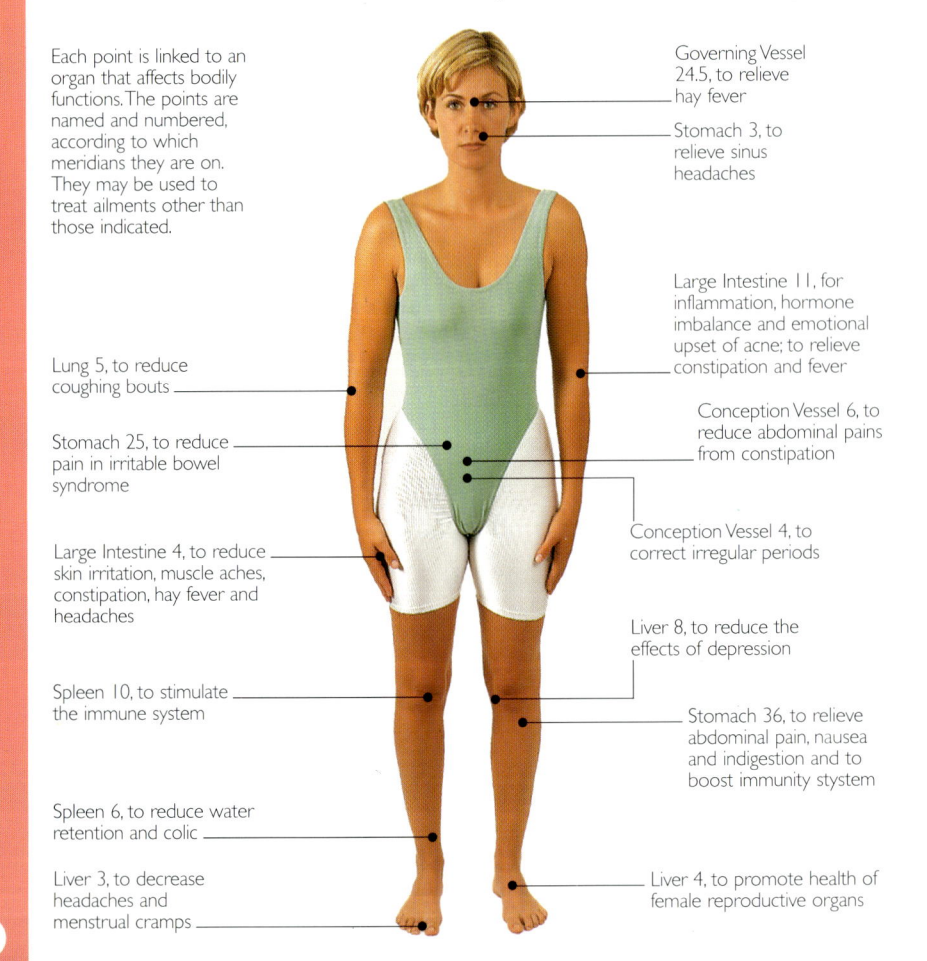

Each point is linked to an organ that affects bodily functions. The points are named and numbered, according to which meridians they are on. They may be used to treat ailments other than those indicated.

Lung 5, to reduce coughing bouts

Stomach 25, to reduce pain in irritable bowel syndrome

Large Intestine 4, to reduce skin irritation, muscle aches, constipation, hay fever and headaches

Spleen 10, to stimulate the immune system

Spleen 6, to reduce water retention and colic

Liver 3, to decrease headaches and menstrual cramps

Governing Vessel 24.5, to relieve hay fever

Stomach 3, to relieve sinus headaches

Large Intestine 11, for inflammation, hormone imbalance and emotional upset of acne; to relieve constipation and fever

Conception Vessel 6, to reduce abdominal pains from constipation

Conception Vessel 4, to correct irregular periods

Liver 8, to reduce the effects of depression

Stomach 36, to relieve abdominal pain, nausea and indigestion and to boost immunity system

Liver 4, to promote health of female reproductive organs

What to expect from a practitioner
The therapist will ask a series of questions to find out about your general health, diet and lifestyle. You'll then be asked to sit or lie down on a table or mattress so that the practitioner can proceed with the therapy. There are several techniques, and they differ in the combination of points used and the way the pressure is applied. Massage is typically used during the procedure.

Can i treat myself?
Many of the points for common symptoms can be used at home. Be careful that you don't overstimulate the point because this may cause a worsening of the symptoms for a short period.

> **Warning!**
> Never apply pressure to the abdomen or on Spleen 6 or Large Intestine 4 if you are pregnant.
>
> Do not apply pressure where there is an open wound, infected or inflamed skin, tumour, varicose vein, a possible broken bone or near a recent surgical scar.

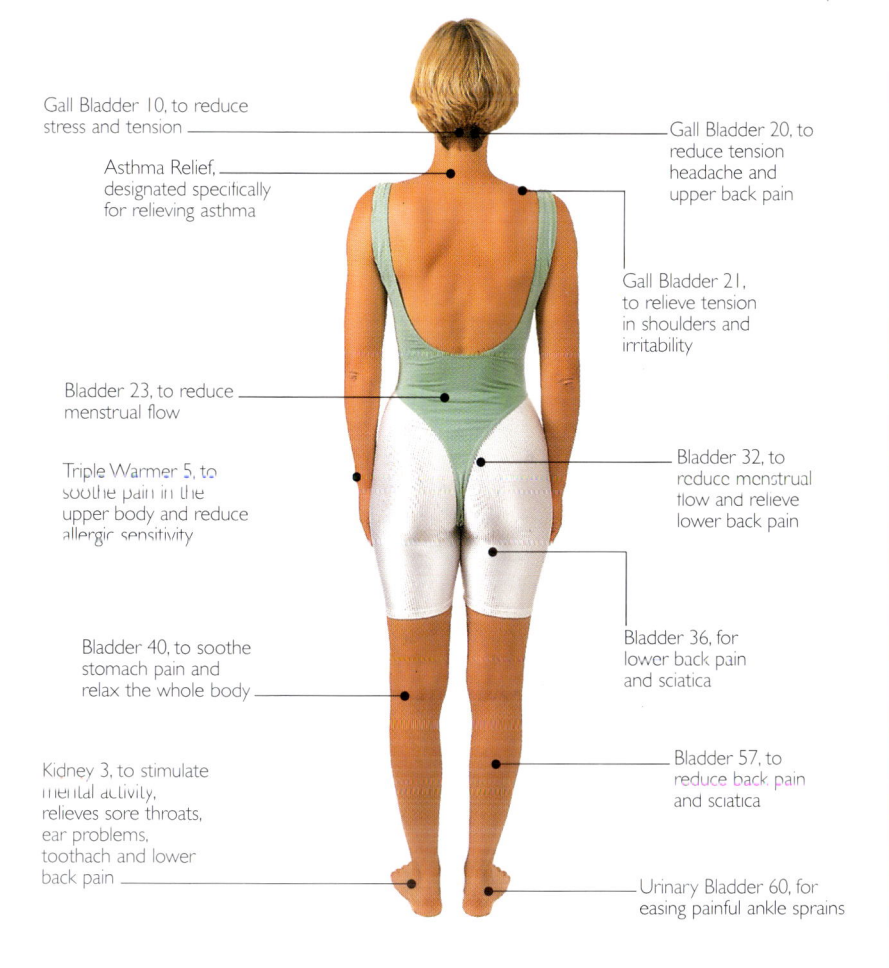

Gall Bladder 10, to reduce stress and tension

Asthma Relief, designated specifically for relieving asthma

Gall Bladder 20, to reduce tension headache and upper back pain

Gall Bladder 21, to relieve tension in shoulders and irritability

Bladder 23, to reduce menstrual flow

Triple Warmer 5, to soothe pain in the upper body and reduce allergic sensitivity

Bladder 32, to reduce menstrual flow and relieve lower back pain

Bladder 40, to soothe stomach pain and relax the whole body

Bladder 36, for lower back pain and sciatica

Kidney 3, to stimulate mental activity, relieves sore throats, ear problems, toothach and lower back pain

Bladder 57, to reduce back pain and sciatica

Urinary Bladder 60, for easing painful ankle sprains

REFLEXOLOGY

APPLYING PRESSURE TO THE POINT

Always use your thumb to put pressure on a reflex point. Bend the thumb first and keep it bent. Using the tip of your thumb – not the nail – press on the point for about a minute, then gently release the pressure without unbending your thumb. If you are doing a series of points, move on to the next point, keeping your thumb bent and as close to the foot as possible.

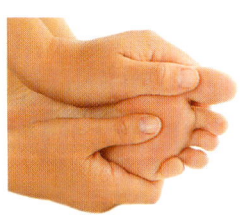

Support the foot with one hand while the other hand is massaging and applying the pressure. Always hold the foot firmly but comfortably.

Warning!
Never have reflexology on your feet if you suffer from thrombosis.

See a practitioner if you have diabetes; don't try reflexology techniques on your feet on your own.

How it works
This type of foot massage that concentrates on specific areas of the feet to treat certain medical conditions is known as reflexology, or zone therapy. Based on similar theories found in traditional Chinese treatments, reflexology works on the principle that energy from the entire body flows to the feet. If this energy becomes blocked, it can have an effect on the health of the body.

Although similar foot therapies have been used by other cultures in the past, reflexology is basically a modern treatment – it was developed in the early 20th century by an American physician, Dr William Fitzgerald. He created maps of the feet, showing the areas that correspond with parts of the body. For example, sections of the big toe represent the head and brain. Following Fitzgerald's theory, it is possible to reduce pain from a headache by applying reflexology techniques to the big toe. Reflexology points are also found on the hands, but these are not considered as effective as those on the feet.

What to expect from a practitioner
On your first visit to a reflexologist, you will be asked questions relating to your general health and lifestyle. Leading a busy, stressful life can affect your overall health. While reflexology cannot take the stress out of your life, treatment can help you feel more relaxed.

You'll be asked to sit in a comfortable, reclining position that will allow the reflexologist to work on your feet. The soles of your feet will be examined and may be given a general massage with talcum powder to determine if there are tender and painful areas that need treatment. Treatment will then begin, with the reflexologist firmly but gently manipulating and stroking the feet, using both fingers and thumbs. It is not a painful process, but there may be momentary discomfort when the affected area is first stroked. Several points will be treated on both feet.

Can I treat myself?
It can be difficult to reach some of the points yourself, but you can use those you can reach to treat minor symptoms and conditions.

REFLEXOLOGY POINTS ON THE FEET

In many instances, there are matching points on both your feet. The points on your right foot are said to match the parts on the right side of your body; the ones on your left foot are said to correspond to those on your left side. There are several points, however, that can be found on only one foot, such as the ones for the heart, spleen and gall bladder.

1 Brain/top of head
2 Sinuses/brain/top of head
3 Side of brain and head/neck
4 Pituitary gland
5 Spine
6 Neck/throat/thyroid gland
7 Parathyroid gland
8 Thyroid gland
9 Trachea
10 Eye
11 Eustachian tube
12 Ear
13 Shoulder
14 Lung
15 Heart
16 Solar plexus
17 Stomach
18 Pancreas
19 Kidney
20 Liver
21 Gall bladder
22 Spleen
23 Ascending colon
24 Descending colon
25 Small intestine
26 Bladder
27 Sciatic nerve

RIGHT FOOT

LEFT FOOT

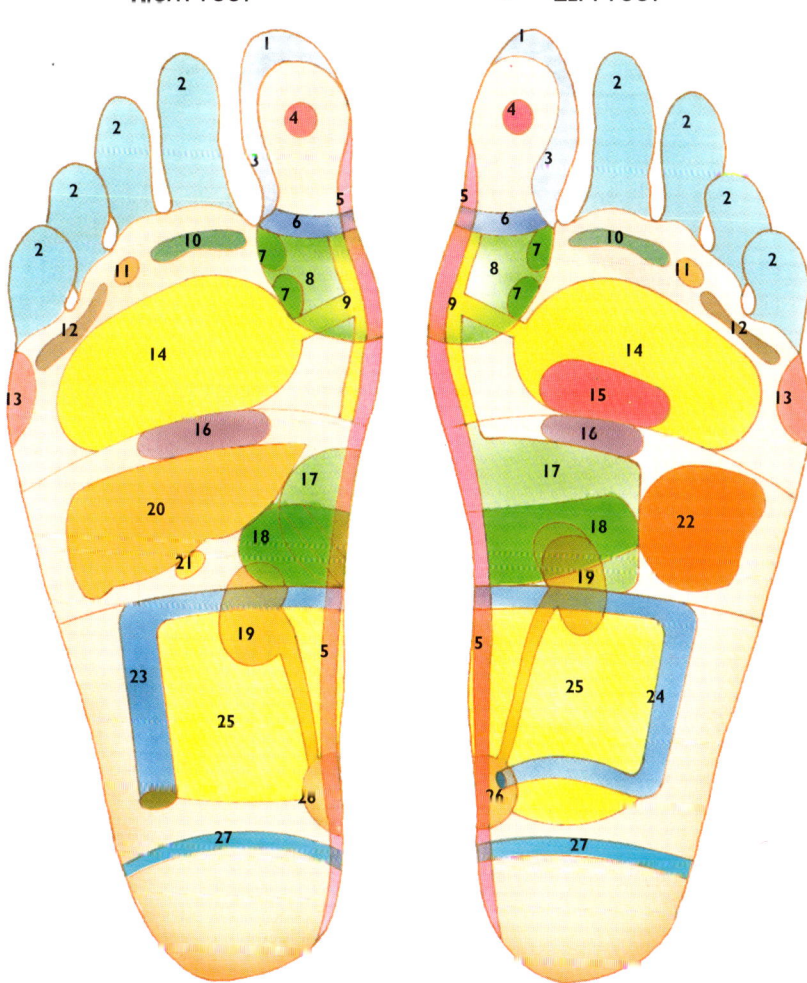

Relaxation & Visualization

Relaxing at Work

It is important to release muscle tension at work – you'll both feel and perform better. Take a few minutes to do some stretching exercises, such as standing and stretching your arms to the ceiling, then to your toes, or stretching your arms behind your back. Even getting up and walking about for a few minutes can help.

How relaxation works

True relaxation is not simply a case of stopping work for the evening. You have to take time to do it correctly. There are many health benefits to be had from relaxing properly, particularly in terms of relieving stress, which can lead to various health problems, such as digestive upsets, and even heart disease. Other conditions that relaxation techniques can help include:

- Pain
- Asthma
- Anxiety
- Nausea

Deep breathing is one way to reduce stress and is essential for relaxation. In fact, breathing exercises are an important part of the ancient traditions of yoga and meditation. Taking only a few minutes a day for breathing exercises is all that's needed. ▶

Breathing exercises for relaxing

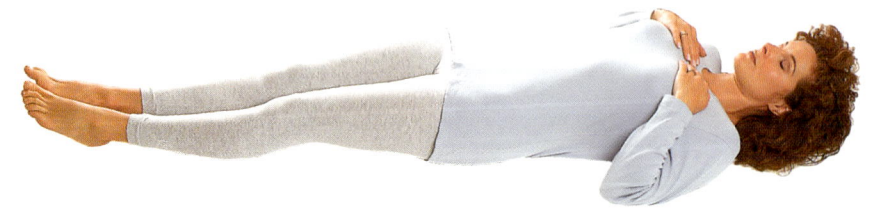

Chest breathing brings oxygen into the lungs quickly and is how we breathe when exercising or in a stressful situation. The exercise is a quick way to help you wake up in the morning and feel more alert when your energy is flagging.

Start by wearing comfortable clothes and removing any footwear. Lie on a comfortable firm surface, with your hands resting gently on your chest and close your eyes. Using the muscles in your chest, slowly breathe in and out. Your hands should rise when you breathe in and fall when you breathe out.

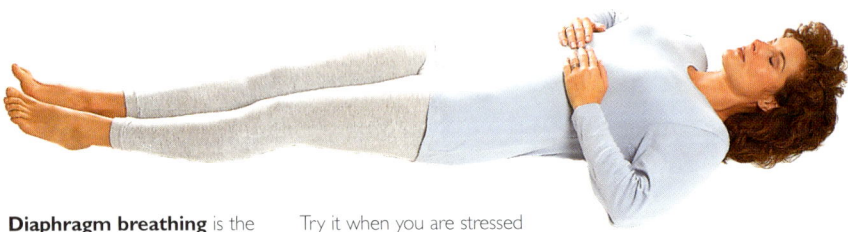

Diaphragm breathing is the natural way to breathe when you are relaxed. It brings more oxygen into the lungs than chest breathing does. It often has to be relearned by adults. Try it when you are stressed or tired.

Lying comfortably on the floor with your eyes closed, place your hands on your abdomen just below your rib cage and breathe in slowly. Feel your hands rising, then breathe out and feel them fall.

How visualization works

Visualization is a form of deep relaxation in which a person tries to imagine certain scenes vividly. It is believed to be helpful for a variety of complaints, including panic and anxiety disorders, heart problems and digestive disorders.

How do I do it?

Begin by sitting or lying comfortably somewhere that you know will be quiet for at least 15 minutes. As you get better at it you may be able to practise visualization anywhere, even in stressful situations. There are two types: external and internal visualization.

- External visualization involves conjuring up images of things, for example, imagining that you are in a beautiful place or somewhere that you were particularly happy, such as an isolated sunny beach on holiday. Use your imagination to picture what is around you, including colours and textures. Try to imagine any smells that may be associated with the scene. Playing relaxing music can add to the atmosphere.
- Internal visualization concentrates on imagining what is going on inside your own body to help it release muscle tension. Each group of muscles is tensed and then relaxed from head to toe. This is one of the best ways to reduce stress.

WHAT ELSE CAN I DO?

There are many other effective ways to relax, and what you do depends on your preferences.
- Exercise, especially swimming, is a good form of relaxation for many people.
- You can relax at home by making sure you unplug the phone and not attempting to do any household duties for an hour.
- Gardening, reading or soaking in a bath are all good ways to unwind.

Internal visualization exercise

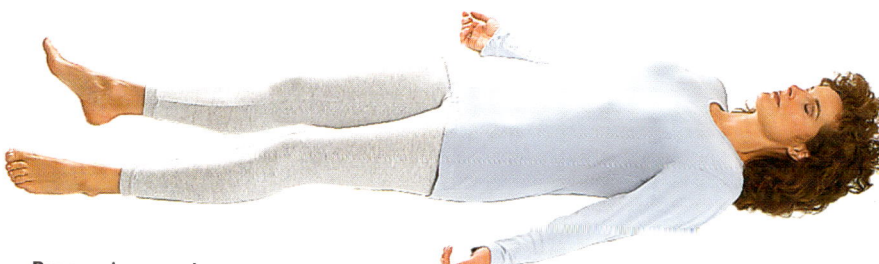

Progressive muscle relaxation releases stress. Lie comfortably on the floor, with your eyes closed, and take deep breaths from your diaphragm (see opposite). Tense each of the muscle groups for a count of 5 and then relax them.

Start with your eyebrows and forehead. For your jaw and face, open your mouth as wide as you can; then tense your neck and shoulder muscles. Lift your arms and tense them;

then tense your rib and stomach muscles. One at a time, raise your legs and tense them and your feet, then gently drop them. Now imagine yourself in a quiet place.

INDEX

A
acne 64–5
acupressure 106–7
allergies 30–1, skin 66–7
anal bleeding 36, 37
anaphylactic shock 30, 59
anxiety 76, 96, 98
aromatherapy 104–5
arthritis 49, 50–1, 52, 54
asthma 22–3
athlete's foot 71

B
back pain 48–9, 54–5
 in pregnancy 80–1
 back strain 42–3
bites, insect 59, 60
blackheads 64–5
bladder problems 74
bleeding 6
 anal 36, 37
 blisters 62
 boils 70
 bowel problems 6, 32–3, 34–5, 38–9
breasts, sore 80–1
breathing exercises 110
breathing problems 6
 see also asthma; bronchitis; panic attacks
bronchitis 24
bruises 58
bursitis 44

C
calluses 69
carbuncles 70
chickenpox 86
chilblains 62
chronic fatigue syndrome 56
colds 18–19
cold sores 15, 76
colic 85
conjunctivitis 12
constipation 34–5
corns 69
coughs 6, 18, 19, 22, 24
"crabs" 72
cradle cap 66, 84
cramp, muscle 46
cuts 58
cysts 64

D, E
dandruff 66, 72
dehydration 33
depression 94–5, 98
dermatitis 66–7
diarrhoea 32–3
disc pain 48–9
dysthymia 94
E. coli bacteria 40
earache 10–11
eczema 66–7
endometriosis 79
eye problems 12–13

F, G
fear 96, 97
fevers 19
fibroids 79
fibrositis 47, 48
flatulence 26, 27
flu 18–19
food: cravings 76, 98
 intolerance 30–1
 poisoning 29, 32, 40
German measles 87
gingivitis 14
gout 53
gums, bleeding 14

H
haemorrhoids 36–7
hay fever 16
headaches 8–9
heartburn 26, 80, 81
herbs 102–3
hiccups 27
homeopathy 100–1
hormone replacement therapy (HRT) 83
hot flushes 82
hydrotherapy 55

I
indigestion 6, 26
insect bites 59, 60
insomnia 92–3
irritable bowel 38–9
itching 66–7, 68
 vaginal 75

L, M
laryngitis 21
lice 72
ligaments, torn 42–3
lumbago 48–9
lyme disease 59
ME see chronic fatigue syndrome
measles 87
menopause 82–3
menstrual cramps 78
migraines 8–9, 28
moles 6
motion sickness 28, 29
mouth ulcers 15
mumps 86

N, O
nappy rash 84
nausea see sickness
neck pain 47
nettle rash 60
nosebleeds 17
obsessive–compulsive disorders 96
oils, essential 104, 105
osteoporosis 82, 83

P
pain, chronic 54–5
panic attacks 96, 97
periods 78, 79
phobias 96
piles 36–7
pregnancy 80–1
premenstrual syndrome 76–7
psoriasis 68

R
rashes 59, 60, 66, 86, 87
rashes, nappy 84
reflexology 108–9
relaxation 110, 111
repetitive strain injury 45
ringworm 71
rubella 87

S
salmonella 40
scabies 71
sciatica 48–9
seasonal affective disorder (SAD) 98
shingles 61
shock 30, 59
shoulder pain 47
sickness 28–9
 "morning" 80, 81
sinusitis 8–9, 17
sleep problems 92–3
spots 64–5, 76
sprains 42–3
stings 59, 60
stomachache 29
strains 42–3, 45
stress 8, 26, 76, 90–1
styes 13
sunburn 63

T
teething problems 88
tendinitis 42–3
TENS machine 55
throats, sore 20–1
thrush 75
tonsillitis 21
toothache 14
travel sickness 28–9

U, V, W
urine problems 6, 74
urticaria 60
verrucas 70
visualization 111
vomiting 26, 28–9, 40
warts 70
water retention 76–7
wind 26, 27, 38

ACKNOWLEDGMENTS

l = left; r = right; b = bottom; t = top; c = centre
All illustrations by Mike Saunders except: p. 12-13, Rudi Vizi. All photographs by Iain Bagwell except: pp. 22bl, 47, 81, 94bl, Andrew Sydenham; p. 81ltr, Laura Wickenden. The publishers would like to thank the Chelsea Physic Garden for supplying the plants shown on pp 11, 13, 25, 32, 36l, 57b, 62, 68, 74, 76, 79, 82, 83, 87, 93; and Gregory Bottley Lloyd for the minerals shown on pp 13r, 57t, 61, 64.